MENOPAUSE VEGAN DIET COOKBOOK

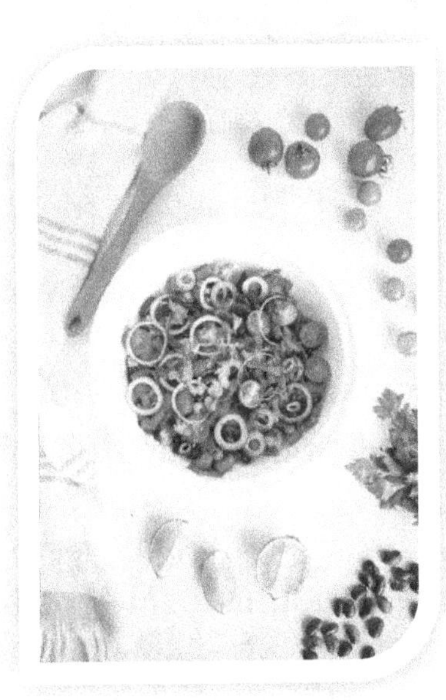

The Ultimate Nutrition Guide with Plant Based Recipes for Natural Management of Menopausal Symptoms

DR.LINDA MCDANIEL

TABLE OF CONTENT

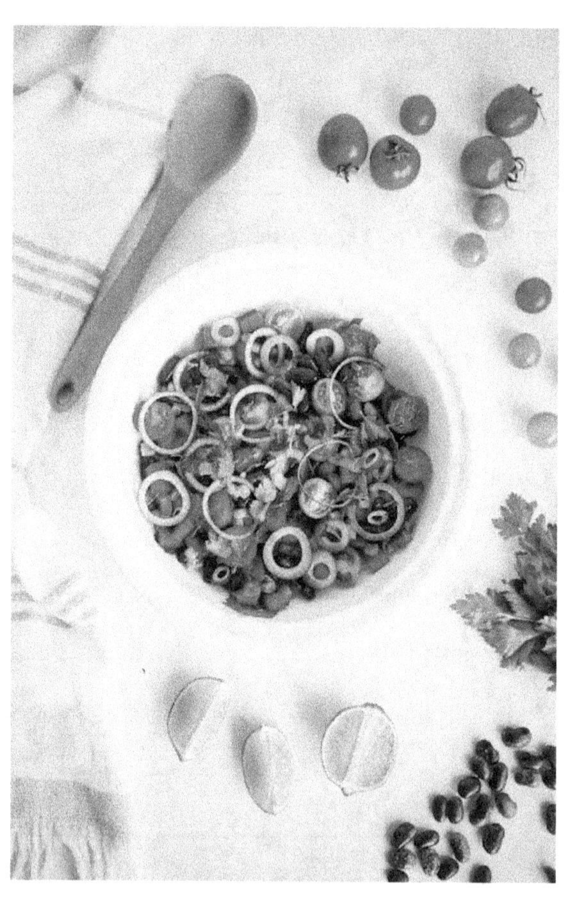

Welcome to the Menopause Vegan Diet Cookbook, a holistic guide crafted with expertise and compassion to support you through the transformative journey of menopause. As a seasoned nutritionist, I understand the profound impact that dietary choices can have on one's well-being, particularly during this pivotal phase of life. With years of experience and a passion for empowering individuals to embrace vibrant health, I am thrilled to share with you a collection of nutritious, flavorful, and anti-inflammatory recipes specifically tailored to address the unique needs of menopausal women.

Menopause is a natural and inevitable transition, yet it can present a myriad of challenges, from hot flashes and mood swings to weight fluctuations and disrupted sleep. However, I firmly believe that through mindful nourishment, we can harness the power of food to alleviate symptoms, promote hormonal balance, and enhance overall vitality.

That's where the Menopause Vegan Diet Cookbook comes in – a comprehensive resource designed to equip you with the tools and knowledge needed to navigate this transformative time with grace and resilience.

In these pages, you'll discover a treasure trove of plant-based recipes thoughtfully curated to nourish your body, soothe inflammation, and ignite your taste buds. From vibrant salads bursting with nutrients to comforting soups infused with healing herbs and spices, each dish is not only delicious but also packed with ingredients specifically chosen to support hormonal health and promote optimal well-being.

But this cookbook is more than just a collection of recipes – it's a roadmap to holistic health and vitality. Throughout these pages, you'll find invaluable insights into the science behind menopause and the role that nutrition plays in mitigating its effects. You'll learn about the anti-inflammatory properties of certain foods, the importance of balancing hormones through diet, and practical tips for incorporating more plant-based meals into your lifestyle.

Whether you're embarking on your menopausal journey or seeking to support a loved one through this transition, the Menopause Vegan Diet Cookbook is your trusted companion on the path to wellness. With each recipe, you're not just nourishing your body – you're nourishing your soul, reclaiming your vitality, and embracing the beauty of menopause as a new chapter in your life's journey.

So, join me as we embark on this delicious adventure together. Let's harness the power of plant-based nutrition to thrive during menopause and beyond. Here's to vibrant health, delicious meals, and a future filled with vitality!

With warmth and gratitude,

Dr. Linda McDaniel Nutritionist and Author

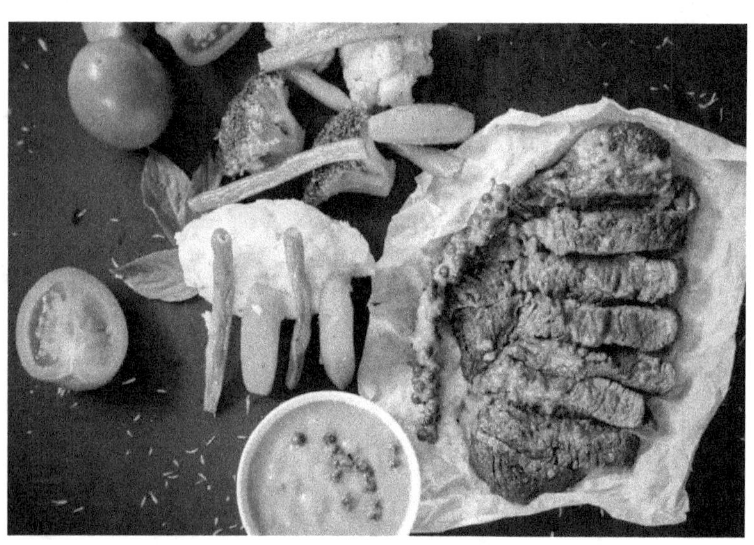

CHAPTER 1:

Understanding the Transition and Empowering Wellness

Menopause is a natural biological process marking the end of a woman's reproductive years. It typically occurs in women between the ages of 45 and 55, although the exact timing can vary widely among individuals. This transformative phase is characterized by a decline in hormone production, particularly estrogen and progesterone, leading to the cessation of menstruation and the end of fertility. While menopause is a universal experience for women, its effects can vary widely, impacting physical, emotional, and psychological well-being.

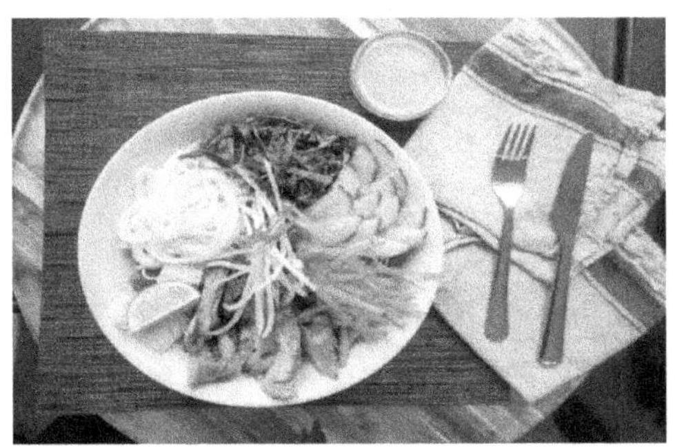

Types of Menopause

There are several types of menopause, each with its own unique characteristics:

1. **Natural Menopause:** This is the most common type of menopause and occurs when a woman's ovaries gradually decrease their production of reproductive hormones, leading to the cessation of menstruation. Natural menopause is typically a gradual process, with symptoms appearing over several years.

2. **Surgical Menopause:** Surgical menopause occurs when a woman's ovaries are surgically removed, either as part of a hysterectomy (removal of the uterus) or oophorectomy (removal of the ovaries). In this case, menopause symptoms can be more sudden and severe due to the abrupt cessation of hormone production.

3. **Premature Menopause:** Premature menopause, also known as early menopause, occurs when menopause begins before the age of 40.

This can be caused by various factors, including genetics, autoimmune disorders, certain medical treatments such as chemotherapy or radiation therapy, or surgical removal of the ovaries.

Causes of Menopause

The primary cause of menopause is the natural aging process, which leads to a decline in ovarian function and hormone production. As women approach their late 30s and early 40s, the number of follicles (structures within the ovaries that contain eggs) begins to decline, leading to a decrease in estrogen and progesterone levels. Eventually, the ovaries stop releasing eggs altogether, resulting in the end of menstruation and the onset of menopause.

Symptoms of Menopause

Menopause is associated with a wide range of symptoms, which can vary in severity from woman to woman. Some common symptoms include:

1. **Hot Flashes:** Sudden, intense feelings of heat, often accompanied by sweating and flushing of the skin.

2. **Night Sweats:** Episodes of excessive sweating during sleep, which can disrupt sleep patterns and lead to fatigue.

3. **Mood Swings:** Emotional fluctuations, including irritability, anxiety, and depression.

4. **Vaginal Dryness:** Decreased lubrication in the vaginal area, leading to discomfort or pain during intercourse.

5. **Changes in Libido:** Decreased interest in sexual activity or changes in sexual function.

6. **Sleep Disturbances:** Difficulty falling asleep or staying asleep, often due to night sweats or hormonal fluctuations.

7. **Weight Gain:** Changes in metabolism and hormone levels can lead to weight gain, particularly around the abdomen.

8. **Bone Loss:** Decreased estrogen levels can contribute to bone loss and an increased risk of osteoporosis.

While menopause is a natural and unavoidable process, there are several preventive measures that women can take to manage symptoms and promote overall well-being:

1. **Maintain a Healthy Lifestyle:** Eating a balanced diet, exercising regularly, and avoiding smoking and excessive alcohol consumption can help alleviate symptoms and support overall health during menopause.

2. **Hormone Replacement Therapy (HRT):** For women experiencing severe symptoms, hormone replacement therapy may be recommended to supplement declining hormone levels and alleviate symptoms such as hot flashes and vaginal dryness. However, HRT carries certain risks and should be discussed with a healthcare provider.

3. **Manage Stress:** Practicing relaxation techniques such as deep breathing, meditation,

and yoga can help reduce stress levels and alleviate symptoms such as mood swings and sleep disturbances.

4. **Supportive Therapies:** Alternative therapies such as acupuncture, herbal supplements, and biofeedback may provide relief from menopausal symptoms for some women. However, it's important to consult with a qualified healthcare provider before trying any new treatments.

5. **Regular Health Screenings:** As women age, regular health screenings become increasingly important for detecting and managing conditions such as osteoporosis, heart disease, and certain cancers. Be sure to schedule regular check-ups with your healthcare provider and discuss any concerns or symptoms you may be experiencing.

In conclusion, menopause is a natural and inevitable transition that marks the end of a woman's reproductive years. While it can be accompanied by a variety of symptoms and challenges, there are many preventive measures and treatment options available to help women manage symptoms and maintain overall health and well-being during this transformative phase of life.

CHAPTER 2

Benefit of Following Menopause Vegan Diet

Adopting a Menopause Vegan Diet can be a powerful way to support optimal health during this transformative phase of life. By focusing on nutrient-rich plant-based foods and avoiding certain dietary triggers, women can effectively manage menopausal symptoms and promote overall well-being.

Foods to Eat:

1. **Whole Grains:** Incorporate whole grains such as quinoa, brown rice, oats, and barley into your diet to provide sustained energy and support digestive health.

2. **Fruits and Vegetables:** Load up on a variety of colorful fruits and vegetables, which are rich in vitamins, minerals, and antioxidants. Aim for a diverse range of produce to ensure you're getting a wide array of nutrients.

3. Legumes: Beans, lentils, and chickpeas are excellent sources of protein, fiber, and phytonutrients. They can help stabilize blood sugar levels, promote satiety, and support hormonal balance.

4. Nuts and Seeds: Include a variety of nuts and seeds such as almonds, walnuts, chia seeds, and flaxseeds in your diet for healthy fats, protein, and essential nutrients like omega-3 fatty acids.

5. Plant-Based Protein: Incorporate tofu, tempeh, edamame, and other plant-based protein sources to meet your daily protein needs and support muscle health.

6. Healthy Fats: Choose sources of healthy fats such as avocados, olives, and coconut oil to support brain function, hormone production, and cardiovascular health.

Foods to Avoid:

1. Processed Foods: Minimize your intake of processed and packaged foods, which often contain additives, preservatives, and excess sodium that can contribute to inflammation and worsen menopausal symptoms.

2. **Sugary Foods and Beverages:** Limit your consumption of sugary snacks, desserts, and sugary beverages like soda and sweetened juices. Excess sugar can disrupt blood sugar levels and contribute to weight gain.

3. **Caffeine and Alcohol:** While moderate consumption of caffeine and alcohol may be acceptable for some women, excessive intake can disrupt sleep patterns, exacerbate hot flashes, and contribute to mood swings. Opt for herbal teas and alcohol-free beverages as alternatives.

4. **High-Sodium Foods:** Reduce your intake of high-sodium foods such as processed meats, canned soups, and salty snacks, as excess sodium can contribute to bloating, water retention, and high blood pressure.

5. **Spicy Foods:** Some women find that spicy foods can trigger hot flashes and exacerbate symptoms. If you're sensitive to spicy foods, consider reducing your intake or opting for milder alternatives.

By focusing on whole, nutrient-dense plant-based foods and minimizing or avoiding processed, sugary, and inflammatory foods, women can optimize their health and well-being during menopause. Remember to listen to your body's cues and make adjustments to your diet as needed to support your individual health goals and preferences.

Complications of Menopause if the right Diet isn't Adopted

Failure to adopt the right diet during menopause can lead to various complications that may impact a woman's health and well-being.

Here are some of the potential complications:

1. **Increased Risk of Chronic Diseases:** Without proper dietary support, women going through menopause may face an increased risk of developing chronic diseases such as heart disease, osteoporosis, and certain types of cancer.

A diet lacking in essential nutrients can contribute to poor cardiovascular health, weakened bones, and impaired immune function, making women more susceptible to these conditions.

2. **Hormonal Imbalance:** Menopause already disrupts hormone levels, and a poor diet can further exacerbate hormonal imbalance. Imbalanced hormone levels can lead to a range of symptoms, including hot flashes, mood swings, and decreased libido. Additionally, hormonal imbalance may increase the risk of conditions such as polycystic ovary syndrome (PCOS) or endometriosis.

3. **Weight Gain and Obesity:** Menopause often coincides with changes in metabolism and body composition, making women more prone to weight gain, particularly around the abdomen. Without proper dietary intervention, unhealthy eating habits can exacerbate weight gain and increase the risk of obesity, which is associated with numerous health complications,

including diabetes, high blood pressure, and heart disease.

4. **Bone Health Complications:** Estrogen plays a crucial role in maintaining bone density, and its decline during menopause can lead to an increased risk of osteoporosis and fractures. A diet lacking in calcium, vitamin D, and other bone-supporting nutrients can further compromise bone health, increasing the likelihood of fractures and other skeletal complications.

5. **Mental Health Issues:** Poor nutrition during menopause can negatively impact mental health, contributing to symptoms such as anxiety, depression, and cognitive decline. Nutrient deficiencies, particularly in omega-3 fatty acids and B vitamins, can impair brain function and exacerbate mood disorders, affecting overall quality of life.

6. **Compromised Immune Function:** A diet lacking in essential nutrients can weaken the immune system, making women more susceptible to infections and illnesses.

This compromised immune function can prolong recovery times and exacerbate menopausal symptoms, further impacting overall health and well-being.

In conclusion, adopting the right diet during menopause is crucial for supporting overall health and minimizing the risk of complications. A nutrient-rich, balanced diet that prioritizes whole foods can help alleviate symptoms, promote hormonal balance, and reduce the risk of chronic diseases, empowering women to navigate this transformative phase of life with vitality and resilience.

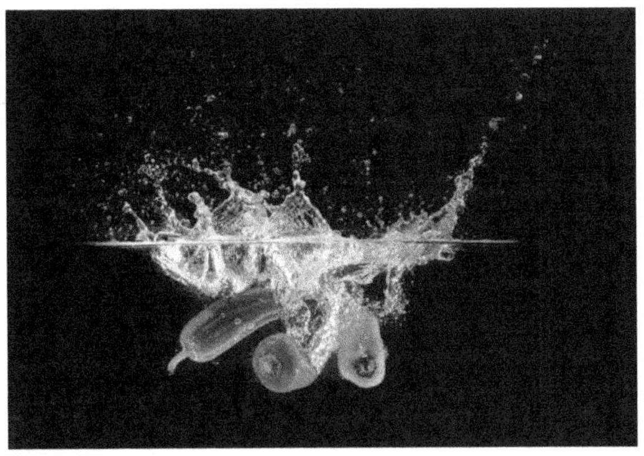

7 DAY MEAL PLAN

Day 1:

Breakfast:

Avocado Toast with Whole Grain Bread topped with sliced avocado, cherry tomatoes, and a sprinkle of nutritional yeast.

Lunch:

Quinoa Salad with mixed greens, cucumber, bell peppers, chickpeas, and a lemon tahini dressing.

Dinner:

Lentil and Vegetable Stir-Fry served over brown rice with broccoli, bell peppers, carrots, and snap peas in a savory ginger-garlic sauce.

Snack:

Sliced apple with almond butter

Day 2:

Breakfast:

Smoothie Bowl topped with blended berries, banana, spinach, and hemp seeds, garnished with granola and sliced almonds.

Lunch:

Mediterranean Chickpea Salad with mixed greens, cherry tomatoes, olives, red onion, and marinated chickpeas, dressed in a lemon herb vinaigrette.

Dinner:

Stuffed Bell Peppers filled with quinoa, black beans, corn, diced tomatoes, and spices, served with a side of steamed green beans.

Snack:

Carrot sticks with hummus.

Day 3:

Breakfast:

Chia Seed Pudding made with almond milk, chia seeds, and vanilla extract, topped with mixed berries and shredded coconut.

Lunch:

Vegan Buddha Bowl with roasted sweet potatoes, kale, black beans, avocado, and tahini drizzle, served over a bed of quinoa.

Dinner:

Spaghetti Squash Pad Thai with tofu, broccoli, carrots, and peanuts in a tangy peanut sauce.

Snack:

Trail mix with raw nuts, seeds, and dried fruit.

Day 4:

Breakfast:

Overnight Oats made with rolled oats, almond milk, chia seeds, and sliced banana, topped with crushed walnuts and a drizzle of maple syrup.

Lunch:

Vegan Greek Salad with romaine lettuce, cucumber, cherry tomatoes, kalamata olives, red onion, and tofu feta, dressed in a lemon-oregano vinaigrette.

Dinner:

Vegetable Curry with cauliflower, potatoes, peas, and spinach in a coconut milk curry sauce, served over brown rice.

Snack:

Sliced mango with lime juice and chili powder.

Day 5:

Breakfast:

Breakfast Burrito filled with scrambled tofu, black beans, avocado, salsa, and spinach, wrapped in a whole grain tortilla.

Lunch:

Quinoa and Black Bean Salad with bell peppers, corn, red onion, cilantro, and lime vinaigrette, served over a bed of mixed greens.

Dinner:

Vegan Lentil Soup with carrots, celery, onions, tomatoes, and kale, seasoned with garlic and thyme.

Snack:

Rice cakes with almond butter and sliced strawberries.

Day 6:

Breakfast:

Green Smoothie made with spinach, kale, banana, pineapple, and coconut water, blended until smooth.

Lunch:

Vegan Taco Salad with mixed greens, black beans, corn, avocado, salsa, and tortilla strips, dressed in a creamy cilantro-lime dressing.

Dinner:

Cauliflower Steak with roasted Brussels sprouts and a balsamic glaze, served with quinoa pilaf.

Snack:

Celery sticks with peanut butter.

Day 7:

Breakfast:

Tofu Scramble with diced bell peppers, onions, and spinach, seasoned with turmeric, garlic powder, and nutritional yeast.

Lunch:

Rainbow Sushi Rolls made with quinoa, avocado, cucumber, bell peppers, and mango, wrapped in nori seaweed and served with soy sauce.

Dinner:

Vegan Chickpea Curry with coconut milk, tomatoes, onions, and garlic, served over basmati rice.

Snack:

Frozen grapes

CHAPTER 3

Menopause Vegan Diet Recipes

Energizing Breakfast:

1. Avocado Toast

Ingredients:

2 slices of whole grain bread

1 ripe avocado

Cherry tomatoes, sliced

Nutritional yeast

Preparation:

1. Toast the bread slices until golden brown.
2. Mash the avocado and spread it evenly on the toast.
3. Top with sliced cherry tomatoes and a sprinkle of nutritional yeast.

Nutritional Value (per serving): Calories: 250, Protein: 7g, Carbohydrates: 25g, Fat: 15g

Cooking Time: 5 minutes

2. Berry Chia Seed Pudding

Ingredients:

1/4 cup chia seeds

1 cup unsweetened almond milk

1/2 teaspoon vanilla extract

Mixed berries (strawberries, blueberries, raspberries)

Preparation:

1. In a bowl, mix chia seeds, almond milk, and vanilla extract. Stir well and let it sit for 10 minutes.

2. Stir the mixture again to prevent clumping. Refrigerate for at least 2 hours or overnight.

3. Serve topped with mixed berries.

Nutritional Value (per serving): Calories: 180, Protein: 6g, Carbohydrates: 20g, Fat: 9g

Cooking Time: 10 minutes (+ refrigeration time)

3. Tofu Scramble

Ingredients:

- 200g firm tofu, crumbled

- 1/2 cup chopped bell peppers

- 1/4 cup diced onions

- 1 cup spinach leaves

- 1/2 teaspoon turmeric

- 1/2 teaspoon garlic powder

- Salt and pepper to taste

Preparation:

1. Heat a non-stick skillet over medium heat. Add onions and bell peppers, sauté until softened.

2. Add crumbled tofu, turmeric, garlic powder, salt, and pepper. Cook for 5-7 minutes, stirring occasionally.

3. Add spinach leaves and cook until wilted and Serve hot.

Nutritional Value (per serving): Calories: 180, Protein: 15g, Carbohydrates: 8g, Fat: 10g
Cooking Time: 15 minutes

4. Quinoa Breakfast Bowl

Ingredients:

- 1/2 cup cooked quinoa

- 1/4 cup almond milk

- 1 tablespoon maple syrup

- 1/4 teaspoon cinnamon

- Sliced banana

- Chopped nuts (walnuts, almonds)

Preparation:

1. In a saucepan, heat almond milk, maple syrup, and cinnamon until warm.

2. Stir in cooked quinoa until well combined.

3. Transfer to a bowl and top with sliced banana and chopped nuts.

Nutritional Value (per serving): Calories: 280, Protein: 7g, Carbohydrates: 40g, Fat: 10g

Cooking Time: 10 minutes

5. Green Smoothie Bowl

Ingredients:

- 1 cup spinach leaves

- 1/2 cup kale leaves

- 1/2 frozen banana

- 1/2 cup frozen mixed berries

- 1/2 cup unsweetened almond milk

- 1 tablespoon chia seeds

Preparation:

1. In a blender, combine spinach, kale, banana, berries, and almond milk. Blend until smooth.

2. Pour into a bowl and sprinkle chia seeds on top.

3. Garnish with additional berries or sliced fruit if desired.

Nutritional Value (per serving): Calories: 200, Protein: 6g, Carbohydrates: 30g, Fat: 8g

Cooking Time: 5 minutes

6. Oatmeal with Almond Butter

Ingredients:

- 1/2 cup rolled oats

- 1 cup water or almond milk

- 1 tablespoon almond butter

- Sliced banana

- Drizzle of maple syrup (optional)

Preparation:

1. In a saucepan, bring water or almond milk to a boil.

2. Stir in rolled oats and reduce heat to simmer. Cook until oats are creamy, about 5 minutes.

3. Transfer to a bowl and top with almond butter, sliced banana, and a drizzle of maple syrup if desired.

Nutritional Value (per serving): Calories: 300, Protein: 9g, Carbohydrates: 40g, Fat: 10g

Cooking Time: 10 minutes

7. Coconut Yogurt Parfait

Ingredients:

- 1 cup unsweetened coconut yogurt

- 1/4 cup granola

- Mixed berries (strawberries, blueberries, raspberries)

- Shredded coconut

Preparation:

1. In a glass or jar, layer coconut yogurt, granola, and mixed berries.

2. Repeat layers until the jar is filled.

3. Top with shredded coconut.

   Nutritional Value (per serving):

   Calories: 250, Protein: 6g, Carbohydrates: 30g, Fat: 12g

   Cooking Time: 5 minutes

8. Banana Walnut Pancakes

Ingredients:

- 1 ripe banana, mashed

- 1/2 cup almond milk

- 1 tablespoon maple syrup

- 1 cup whole wheat flour

- 1 teaspoon baking powder

- 1/4 cup chopped walnuts

Preparation:

1. In a bowl, mix mashed banana, almond milk, and maple syrup until well combined.

2. Add whole wheat flour, baking powder, and chopped walnuts. Stir until just combined.

3. Heat a non-stick skillet over medium heat. Pour batter onto the skillet to form pancakes.

4. Cook until bubbles form on the surface, then flip and cook until golden brown on both sides.

5. Serve hot with maple syrup and additional sliced banana if desired.

Nutritional Value (per serving, 2 pancakes): Calories: 280, Protein: 8g, Carbohydrates: 40g, Fat: 10g

Cooking Time: 15 minutes

9. Vegan Breakfast Burrito

Ingredients:

- 1 whole grain tortilla

- Scrambled tofu (see recipe above)

- Black beans, drained and rinsed

- Salsa

- Sliced avocado

Preparation:

1. Warm the tortilla in a skillet or microwave.

2. Fill the tortilla with scrambled tofu, black beans, salsa, and sliced avocado.

3. Roll up the tortilla into a burrito.

4. Serve hot.

Nutritional Value (per serving):

Calories: 350, Protein: 15g, Carbohydrates: 40g,Fat: 15g

Cooking Time: 10 minutes

10. Vegan Breakfast Sandwich

Ingredients:

- 2 slices of whole grain bread

- Vegan sausage patty

- Sliced tomato

- Baby spinach leaves

- Vegan cheese

Preparation:

1. Cook the vegan sausage patty according to package instructions.

2. Toast the bread slices until golden brown.

3. Assemble the sandwich by layering vegan sausage patty, sliced tomato, baby spinach leaves, and vegan cheese between the toasted bread slices.

4. Optional: Grill the assembled sandwich in a panini press for a crispy exterior and melty cheese and serve hot.

Nutritional Value (per serving): Calories: 350, Protein: 15g, Carbohydrates: 30g, Fat: 15g

Cooking Time: 10 minutes

Ingredients:

- 1 1/2 cups whole wheat flour

- 1 teaspoon baking powder

- 1/2 teaspoon baking soda

- 1/4 teaspoon salt

- 2 ripe bananas, mashed

- 1/4 cup maple syrup

- 1/4 cup unsweetened applesauce

- 1/4 cup almond milk

- 1 teaspoon vanilla extract

- 1 cup fresh or frozen blueberries

Preparation:

1. Preheat the oven to 350°F (175°C). Line a muffin tin with paper liners or lightly grease the cups.

2. In a large bowl, whisk together the whole wheat flour, baking powder, baking soda, and salt.

3. In a separate bowl, mix together the mashed bananas, maple syrup, applesauce, almond milk, and vanilla extract until well combined.

4. Pour the wet ingredients into the dry ingredients and stir until just combined. Be careful not to overmix.

5. Gently fold in the blueberries.

6. Divide the batter evenly among the muffin cups, filling each about two-thirds full.

7. Bake for 20-25 minutes, or until a toothpick inserted into the center of a muffin comes out clean.

8. Allow the muffins to cool in the tin for 5 minutes before transferring to a wire rack to cool completely.

Nutritional Value (per muffin):

Calories: 150, Protein: 3g, Carbohydrates: 30g, Fat: 2g

Cooking Time: 25 minutes

12. Sweet Potato Breakfast Bowl

Ingredients:

- 1 small sweet potato, peeled and diced

- 1/4 teaspoon cinnamon

- 1 tablespoon maple syrup

- 1/4 cup chopped pecans

- 1 tablespoon unsweetened coconut flakes

- Plant-based yogurt (optional)

Preparation:

1. Preheat the oven to 400°F (200°C). Line a baking sheet with parchment paper.

2. In a bowl, toss the diced sweet potato with cinnamon and maple syrup until evenly coated.

3. Spread the sweet potato cubes in a single layer on the prepared baking sheet.

4. Roast in the preheated oven for 20-25 minutes, or until tender and caramelized.

5. In a dry skillet, toast the chopped pecans and coconut flakes until fragrant and lightly browned.

6. To assemble the breakfast bowl, layer the roasted sweet potato cubes with toasted pecans, coconut flakes, and a dollop of plant-based yogurt if desired.

7. Drizzle with additional maple syrup if desired.

Nutritional Value (per serving): Calories: 250, Protein: 4g, Carbohydrates: 35g, Fat: 10g

Cooking Time: 30 minutes

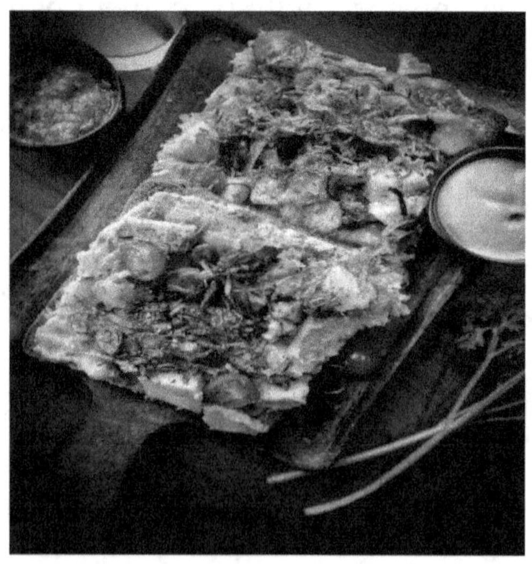

13. Vegan Breakfast Hash

Ingredients:

- 1 tablespoon olive oil

- 1 small onion, diced

- 2 cloves garlic, minced

- 2 cups diced potatoes

- 1 cup diced bell peppers

- 1 cup diced zucchini

- 1 cup cooked chickpeas

- 1 teaspoon smoked paprika

- Salt and pepper to taste

- Fresh parsley for garnish

Preparation:

1. Heat olive oil in a large skillet over medium heat. Add diced onion and garlic, sauté until softened.

2. Add diced potatoes to the skillet and cook until golden brown and crispy, stirring occasionally.

3. Add diced bell peppers, zucchini, and cooked chickpeas to the skillet. Cook until vegetables are tender.

4. Season with smoked paprika, salt, and pepper to taste.

5. Garnish with fresh parsley before serving.

Nutritional Value (per serving): Calories: 300, Protein: 8g, Carbohydrates: 45g, Fat: 10g

Cooking Time: 25 minutes

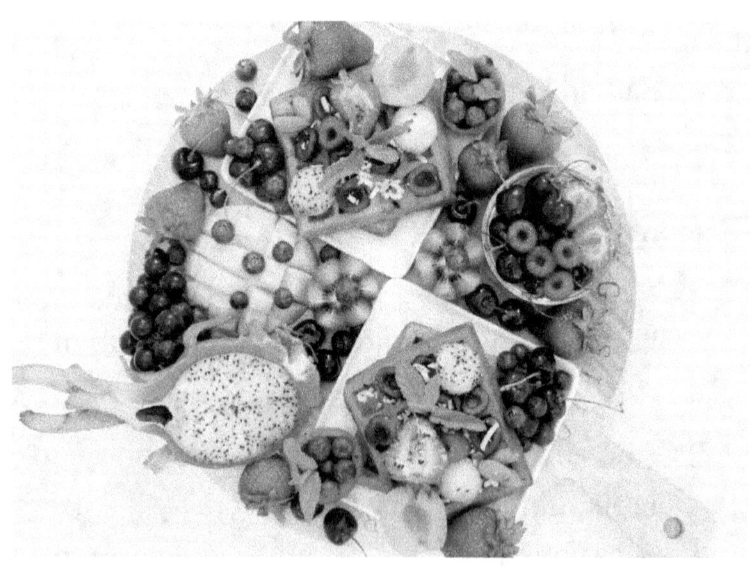

14. Vegan Banana Bread

Ingredients:

- 2 ripe bananas, mashed

- 1/4 cup maple syrup

- 1/4 cup unsweetened applesauce

- 1/4 cup almond milk

- 1 teaspoon vanilla extract

- 1 1/2 cups whole wheat flour

- 1 teaspoon baking powder

- 1/2 teaspoon baking soda

- 1/4 teaspoon salt

- 1/2 cup chopped walnuts (optional)

Preparation:

1. Preheat the oven to 350°F (175°C). Grease a loaf pan or line it with parchment paper.

2. In a large bowl, whisk together the mashed bananas, maple syrup, applesauce,

almond milk, and vanilla extract until well combined.

3. In a separate bowl, sift together the whole wheat flour, baking powder, baking soda, and salt.

4. Gradually add the dry ingredients to the wet ingredients, stirring until just combined. Be careful not to overmix.

5. Fold in the chopped walnuts if using.

6. Pour the batter into the prepared loaf pan and smooth the top with a spatula.

7. Bake in the preheated oven for 45-50 minutes, or until a toothpick inserted into the center of the bread comes out clean.

8. Allow the banana bread to cool in the pan for 10 minutes before transferring it to a wire rack to cool completely.

Nutritional Value (per serving): Calories: 200, Protein: 5g, Carbohydrates: 35g Fat: 7g

Cooking Time: 50 minutes

15. Vegan Breakfast Tacos

Ingredients:

- 4 small whole grain tortillas
- Scrambled tofu (see recipe above)
- Sliced avocado
- Salsa
- Fresh cilantro leaves

Preparation:

1. Warm the tortillas in a skillet or microwave.
2. Fill each tortilla with scrambled tofu, sliced avocado, salsa, and fresh cilantro leaves.
3. Serve hot.

Nutritional Value (per serving, 2 tacos):

- Calories: 300
- Protein: 10g
- Carbohydrates: 25g
- Fat: 15g

Cooking Time: 10 minutes

1. Quinoa Salad with Chickpeas and Lemon Tahini Dressing

Ingredients:

- 1 cup cooked quinoa

- 1/2 cup cooked chickpeas

- Mixed greens

- 1/4 cup diced cucumber

- 1/4 cup diced bell peppers

- Lemon Tahini Dressing (2 tablespoons tahini, juice of 1 lemon, 1 tablespoon water, salt, and pepper)

Preparation:

1. In a bowl, combine cooked quinoa, chickpeas, mixed greens, diced cucumber, and diced bell peppers.

2. In a separate bowl, whisk together tahini, lemon juice, water, salt, and pepper to make the dressing.

3. Drizzle the dressing over the salad and toss until well combined.

Nutritional Value (per serving): Calories: 350, Protein: 10g, Carbohydrates: 45g, Fat: 15g

Cooking Time: 15 minutes

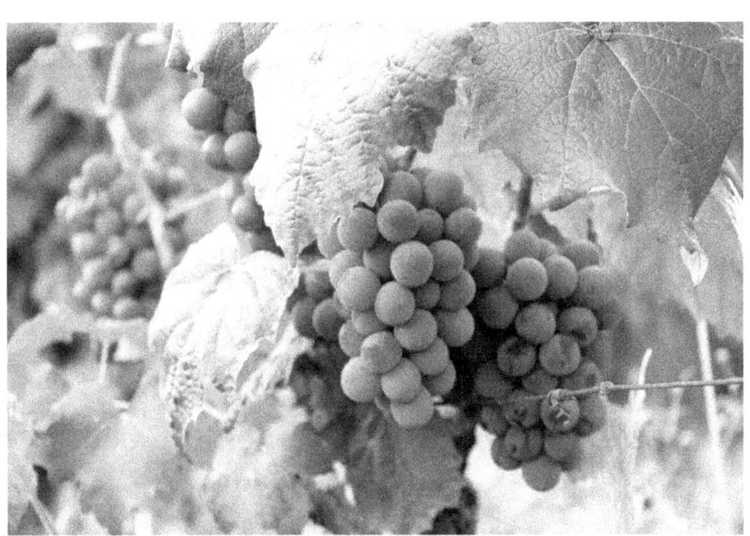

2. Mediterranean Chickpea Salad

Ingredients:

- 1 can (15 oz) chickpeas, drained and rinsed
- Mixed greens
- Cherry tomatoes, halved
- Cucumber, diced
- Red onion, thinly sliced
- Kalamata olives
- Lemon herb vinaigrette (2 tablespoons olive oil, juice of 1 lemon, 1 teaspoon dried oregano, salt, and pepper)

Preparation:

1. In a bowl, combine chickpeas, mixed greens, cherry tomatoes, cucumber, red onion, and Kalamata olives.

2. In a separate bowl, whisk together olive oil, lemon juice, dried oregano, salt, and pepper to make the vinaigrette.

3. Drizzle the vinaigrette over the salad and toss until well coated.

Nutritional Value (per serving): Calories: 300, Protein: 8g, Carbohydrates: 35g, Fat: 15g

Cooking Time: 10 minutes

3. Vegan Buddha Bowl

Ingredients:

- Cooked quinoa or brown rice

- Roasted sweet potatoes

- Steamed broccoli

- Sautéed kale

- Avocado slices

- Lemon tahini dressing (2 tablespoons tahini, juice of 1 lemon, 1 tablespoon water, salt, and pepper)

Preparation:

1. Assemble cooked quinoa or brown rice, roasted sweet potatoes, steamed broccoli, sautéed kale, and avocado slices in a bowl.

2. Drizzle with lemon tahini dressing.

3. Serve warm or at room temperature.

Nutritional Value (per serving): Calories: 400, Protein: 10g, Carbohydrates: 50g, Fat: 20g

Cooking Time: 30 minutes

4. Vegan Greek Salad with Tofu Feta

Ingredients:

- Mixed greens

- Cherry tomatoes, halved

- Cucumber, diced

- Red onion, thinly sliced

- Kalamata olives

- Tofu feta (8 oz firm tofu, crumbled; marinade: 2 tablespoons olive oil, 2 tablespoons lemon juice, 1 teaspoon dried oregano, salt, and pepper)

- Lemon herb vinaigrette (2 tablespoons olive oil, juice of 1 lemon, 1 teaspoon dried oregano, salt, and pepper)

Preparation:

1. In a bowl, combine mixed greens, cherry tomatoes, cucumber, red onion, and Kalamata olives.

2. In a separate bowl, mix together crumbled tofu, olive oil, lemon juice, dried oregano, salt, and pepper to make the tofu feta marinade. Let it marinate for at least 30 minutes.

3. Add tofu feta to the salad and drizzle with lemon herb vinaigrette.

Nutritional Value (per serving): Calories: 350, Protein: 12g, Carbohydrates: 25g, Fat: 20g

Cooking Time: 40 minutes (including marinating time)

5. Vegan Lentil Salad with Balsamic Dressing

Ingredients:

- 1 cup cooked lentils

- Mixed greens

- Cherry tomatoes, halved

- Cucumber, diced

- Red onion, thinly sliced

- Avocado slices

- Balsamic dressing (2 tablespoons balsamic vinegar, 1 tablespoon olive oil, 1 teaspoon Dijon mustard, salt, and pepper)

Preparation:

1. In a bowl, combine cooked lentils, mixed greens, cherry tomatoes, cucumber, red onion, and avocado slices.

2. In a separate bowl, whisk together balsamic vinegar, olive oil, Dijon mustard, salt, and pepper to make the dressing.

3. Drizzle the dressing over the salad and toss until well combined.

Nutritional Value (per serving): Calories: 300, Protein: 10g, Carbohydrates: 35g, Fat: 15g   **Cooking Time: 15 minutes**

6. Vegan Chickpea Curry

Ingredients:

- 1 can (15 oz) chickpeas, drained and rinsed

- 1 cup diced tomatoes

- 1 cup coconut milk

- 1 onion, diced

- 2 cloves garlic, minced

- 1 tablespoon curry powder

- Salt and pepper to taste

- Fresh cilantro for garnish

Preparation:

1. Heat olive oil in a large skillet over medium heat. Add diced onion and garlic, sauté until softened.

2. Add diced tomatoes, chickpeas, coconut milk, curry powder, salt, and pepper to the skillet. Stir to combine.

3. Simmer for 10-15 minutes, stirring occasionally, until the curry has thickened slightly.

4. Serve hot, garnished with fresh cilantro.

Nutritional Value (per serving): Calories: 350, Protein: 12g, Carbohydrates: 30g, Fat: 20g

Cooking Time: 20 minutes

7. Vegan Lentil Soup

Ingredients:

- 1 cup dried green lentils
- 4 cups vegetable broth
- 1 onion, diced
- 2 carrots, diced
- 2 celery stalks, diced
- 2 cloves garlic, minced
- 1 teaspoon dried thyme
- 1 bay leaf
- Salt and pepper to taste
- Fresh parsley for garnish

Preparation:

1. Rinse the lentils under cold water and drain.

2. In a large pot, heat olive oil over medium heat. Add diced onion, carrots, and celery. Sauté until softened.

3. Add minced garlic, dried thyme, and bay leaf. Cook for another minute until fragrant.

4. Pour in vegetable broth and add rinsed lentils to the pot. Bring to a boil, then reduce heat to low and simmer for 20-25 minutes, or until lentils are tender.

5. Season with salt and pepper to taste.

6. Serve hot, garnished with fresh parsley.

Nutritional Value (per serving): Calories: 250, Protein: 15g, Carbohydrates: 40g, Fat: 2g

Cooking Time: 30 minutes

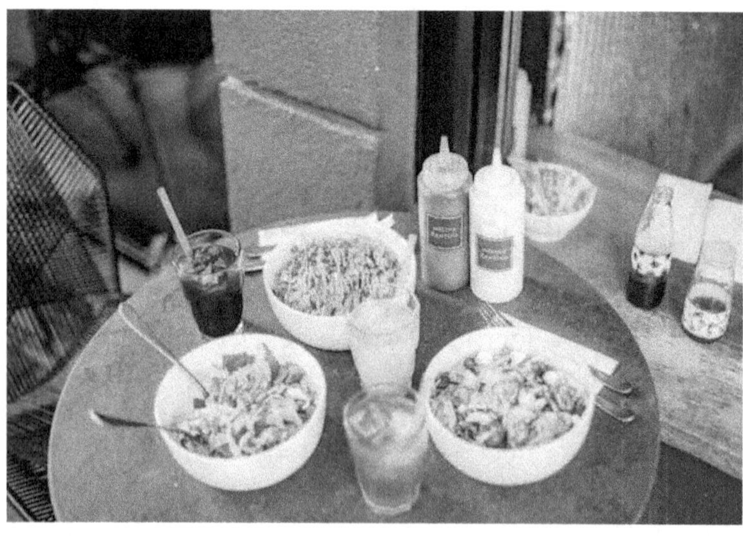

8. Vegan Black Bean Tacos

Ingredients:

- 1 can (15 oz) black beans, drained and rinsed

- Taco shells or tortillas

- Sliced avocado

- Shredded lettuce

- Diced tomatoes

- Salsa

- Fresh cilantro for garnish

Preparation:

1. Heat black beans in a saucepan over medium heat until warmed through.

2. Heat taco shells or tortillas according to package instructions.

3. Assemble tacos with black beans, sliced avocado, shredded lettuce, diced tomatoes, and salsa.

4. Garnish with fresh cilantro.

5. Serve immediately.

Nutritional Value (per serving, 2 tacos): Calories: 300, Protein: 10g, Carbohydrates: 35g, Fat: 15g

Cooking Time: 10 minutes

9. Vegan Vegetable Stir-Fry

Ingredients:

- 2 cups mixed vegetables (broccoli, bell peppers, carrots, snap peas)

- 1 cup cooked quinoa or brown rice

- 1/4 cup low-sodium soy sauce

- 2 cloves garlic, minced

- 1 tablespoon grated ginger

- 1 tablespoon sesame oil

- Sesame seeds for garnish

Preparation:

1. Heat sesame oil in a large skillet or wok over medium heat. Add minced garlic and grated ginger, sauté for 1-2 minutes until fragrant.

2. Add mixed vegetables to the skillet and stir-fry for 5-7 minutes, or until crisp-tender.

3. Pour in low-sodium soy sauce and cooked quinoa or brown rice. Stir to combine and heat through.

4. Garnish with sesame seeds before serving.

Nutritional Value (per serving): Calories: 300, Protein: 10g, Carbohydrates: 45g, Fat: 8g

Cooking Time: 15 minutes

Ingredients:

- 4 bell peppers, halved and seeds removed

- 1 cup cooked quinoa

- 1 can (15 oz) black beans, drained and rinsed

- 1 cup corn kernels

- 1 cup diced tomatoes

- 1 teaspoon chili powder

- 1/2 teaspoon cumin

- Salt and pepper to taste

- Vegan cheese (optional)

- Fresh cilantro for garnish

Preparation:

1. Preheat the oven to 375°F (190°C). Grease a baking dish.

2. In a large bowl, combine cooked quinoa, black beans, corn kernels, diced tomatoes, chili powder, cumin, salt, and pepper.

3. Spoon the quinoa mixture into the halved bell peppers, pressing down gently to pack the filling.

4. If using, sprinkle vegan cheese on top of the stuffed peppers.

5. Place the stuffed peppers in the prepared baking dish and cover with foil.

6. Bake in the preheated oven for 25-30 minutes, or until the peppers are tender.

7. Garnish with fresh cilantro before serving.

Nutritional Value (per serving, 2 pepper halves): Calories: 350, Protein: 15g, Carbohydrates: 45g, Fat: 8g

Cooking Time: 40 minutes

11. Vegan Spaghetti Squash Pad Thai

Ingredients:

- 1 medium spaghetti squash

- 1 cup diced tofu

- 1 cup broccoli florets

- 1 carrot, julienned

- 1/2 cup sliced bell peppers

- 2 cloves garlic, minced

- 1/4 cup chopped peanuts

- Pad Thai sauce (2 tablespoons soy sauce, 1 tablespoon maple syrup, 1 tablespoon lime juice, 1 teaspoon sriracha)

- Fresh cilantro for garnish

Preparation:

1. Preheat the oven to 400°F (200°C). Cut the spaghetti squash in half lengthwise and remove the seeds.

2. Place the squash halves, cut side down, on a baking sheet lined with parchment paper.

Roast in the preheated oven for 40-45 minutes, or until the squash is tender and the flesh can be easily shredded with a fork.

3. While the squash is roasting, prepare the tofu and vegetables. In a large skillet, heat olive oil over medium heat. Add diced tofu and cook until golden brown on all sides. Remove tofu from the skillet and set aside.

4. In the same skillet, add broccoli, carrot, bell peppers, and minced garlic. Sauté until the vegetables are tender-crisp.

5. Use a fork to scrape the flesh of the roasted spaghetti squash into "noodles".

6. Add the spaghetti squash "noodles" and cooked tofu to the skillet with the vegetables.

7. Pour the Pad Thai sauce over the mixture and toss until everything is evenly coated.

8. Serve hot, garnished with chopped peanuts and fresh cilantro.

Nutritional Value (per serving): Calories: 300, Protein: 12g, Carbohydrates: 40g, Fat: 10g

Cooking Time: 60 minutes

12. Vegan Mediterranean Wrap

Ingredients:

- Whole grain tortilla or wrap

- Hummus

- Sliced cucumber

- Sliced tomato

- Mixed greens

- Kalamata olives, sliced

- Sliced red onion

- Lemon herb vinaigrette (2 tablespoons olive oil, juice of 1 lemon, 1 teaspoon dried oregano, salt, and pepper)

Preparation:

1. Spread a generous layer of hummus on the whole grain tortilla or wrap.

2. Layer sliced cucumber, tomato, mixed greens, Kalamata olives, and red onion on top of the hummus.

3. Drizzle with lemon herb vinaigrette.

4. Roll up the tortilla or wrap tightly.

5. Slice in half diagonally before serving.

Nutritional Value (per serving): Calories: 350, Protein: 8g, Carbohydrates: 40g, Fat: 18

Cooking Time: 10 minutes

13. Vegan Lentil Sloppy Joes

Ingredients:

- 1 cup cooked lentils

- 1/2 cup diced onion

- 1/2 cup diced bell peppers

- 1 cup tomato sauce

- 2 tablespoons tomato paste

- 1 tablespoon maple syrup and 1 tablespoon apple cider vinegar

- 1 teaspoon chili powder and 1/2 teaspoon smoked paprika

- Salt and pepper to taste and Whole grain burger buns

Preparation:

1. Heat olive oil in a skillet over medium heat. Add diced onion and bell peppers, sauté until softened.

2. Add cooked lentils, tomato sauce, tomato paste, maple syrup, apple cider vinegar, chili powder, smoked paprika, salt, and pepper to the skillet. Stir to combine.

3. Simmer for 10-15 minutes, stirring occasionally, until the mixture thickens.

4. Serve the lentil mixture on whole grain burger buns.

5. Optionally, serve with sliced pickles or coleslaw on top.

Nutritional Value (per serving): Calories: 300, Protein: 12g, Carbohydrates: 45g, Fat: 5g

Cooking Time: 20 minutes

14. Vegan Falafel Bowl

Ingredients:

- Homemade or store-bought falafel

- Cooked quinoa or brown rice

- Mixed greens

- Sliced cucumber

- Cherry tomatoes, halved

- Tahini sauce (2 tablespoons tahini, juice of 1 lemon, 1 tablespoon water, salt, and pepper)

- Fresh parsley for garnish

Preparation:

1. Prepare falafel according to package instructions or use homemade falafel.

2. Assemble cooked quinoa or brown rice, mixed greens, sliced cucumber, and cherry tomatoes in a bowl.

3. Add falafel to the bowl.

4. Drizzle with tahini sauce.

5. Garnish with fresh parsley.

Nutritional Value (per serving): Calories: 350, Protein: 15g, Carbohydrates: 40g, Fat: 15g

Cooking Time: 30 minutes (if making falafel from scratch)

Ingredients:

- 2 medium sweet potatoes, peeled and diced

- 1 can (15 oz) black beans, drained and rinsed

- 1/2 teaspoon cumin

- 1/2 teaspoon chili powder

- Salt and pepper to taste

- Whole grain tortillas

- Vegan cheese (optional)

- Sliced avocado

- Salsa

Preparation:

1. Steam or boil diced sweet potatoes until tender. Mash with a fork.

2. In a skillet, combine mashed sweet potatoes, black beans, cumin, chili powder, salt, and pepper. Cook until heated through.

3. Heat a separate skillet over medium heat. Place a tortilla in the skillet and spread sweet potato-black bean mixture on half of the tortilla.

4. If using, sprinkle vegan cheese on top of the mixture.

5. Fold the tortilla in half to cover the filling.

6. Cook for 2-3 minutes on each side, until golden brown and crispy.

7. Repeat with remaining tortillas and filling.

8. Serve hot, with sliced avocado and salsa on the side.

Nutritional Value (per serving, 1 quesadilla):

- Calories: 350

- Protein: 10g

- Carbohydrates: 45g

- Fat: 15g

Cooking Time: 30 minutes

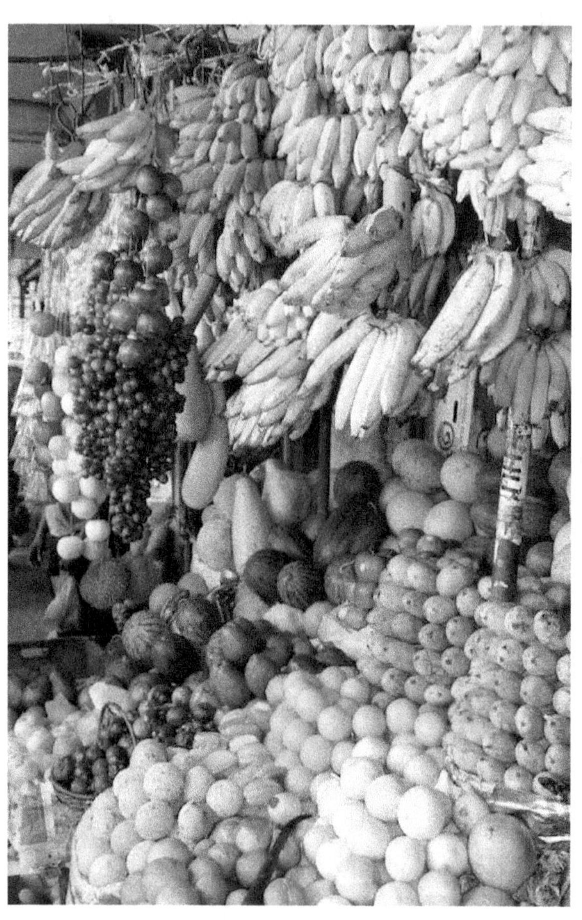

Nourishing Dinner:

1. Vegan Lentil Shepherd's Pie

Ingredients:

- 1 cup dry green lentils & 2 cups vegetable broth

- 2 large potatoes, peeled and diced & 1 tablespoon olive oil

- 1 onion, diced & 2 carrots, diced

- 2 celery stalks, diced & 2 cloves garlic, minced

- 1 cup frozen peas & 1 tablespoon tomato paste

- 1 teaspoon thyme & Salt and pepper to taste

Preparation:

1. Preheat the oven to 375°F (190°C).

2. In a pot, combine lentils and vegetable broth. Bring to a boil, then reduce heat and simmer for 20-25 minutes, until lentils are tender.

3. In a separate pot, boil the diced potatoes until soft. Mash them with a potato masher

or fork, adding a little almond milk or vegetable broth to achieve desired consistency.

4. In a skillet, heat olive oil over medium heat. Add diced onion, carrots, celery, and garlic. Sauté until softened.

5. Add cooked lentils, frozen peas, tomato paste, thyme, salt, and pepper to the skillet. Cook for another 5 minutes.

6. Transfer the lentil mixture to a baking dish. Spread mashed potatoes on top.

7. Bake in the preheated oven for 20-25 minutes, until the top is golden brown.

Nutritional Value (per serving):

- Calories: 350

- Protein: 15g

- Carbohydrates: 60g

- Fat: 5g

Cooking Time: 60 minutes

2. Vegan Chickpea Curry

Ingredients:

- 1 can (15 oz) chickpeas, drained and rinsed & 1 can (14 oz) coconut milk

- 1 onion, diced & 2 cloves garlic, minced

- 1 tablespoon ginger, minced & 2 teaspoons curry powder

- 1 teaspoon turmeric & 1 teaspoon cumin

- Salt and pepper to taste & Fresh cilantro for garnish

Preparation:

1. In a large skillet, heat olive oil over medium heat. Add diced onion, garlic, and ginger. Sauté until softened.

2. Add curry powder, turmeric, and cumin to the skillet. Cook for another minute until fragrant.

3. Add chickpeas and coconut milk to the skillet. Season with salt and pepper.

4. Simmer for 10-15 minutes, until the curry thickens slightly.

5. Serve hot, garnished with fresh cilantro.

Nutritional Value (per serving): Calories: 400, Protein: 15g, Carbohydrates: 45g, Fat: 20g

Cooking Time: 20 minutes

3. Vegan Mushroom Stroganoff

Ingredients:

- 8 oz mushrooms, sliced & 1 onion, diced

- 2 cloves garlic, minced & 1 tablespoon olive oil

- 1 tablespoon flour & 1 cup vegetable broth

- 1/2 cup coconut milk & 2 tablespoons nutritional yeast

- 1 teaspoon Dijon mustard & Salt and pepper to taste

- Cooked pasta or rice & Fresh parsley for garnish

Preparation:

1. In a large skillet, heat olive oil over medium heat. Add sliced mushrooms and diced onion. Sauté until mushrooms are golden brown and onions are translucent.

2. Add minced garlic to the skillet and cook for another minute.

3. Sprinkle flour over the mushrooms and stir to coat.

4. Gradually pour in vegetable broth, stirring constantly to prevent lumps from forming.

5. Stir in coconut milk, nutritional yeast, and Dijon mustard. Cook until the sauce thickens.

6. Season with salt and pepper to taste.

7. Serve over cooked pasta or rice, garnished with fresh parsley.

Nutritional Value (per serving): Calories: 350, Protein: 10g, Carbohydrates: 45g, Fat: 15g

Cooking Time: 30 minutes

Ingredients:

- 1 eggplant, diced & 2 zucchinis, diced

- 1 bell pepper, diced & 1 onion, diced

- 2 cloves garlic, minced & 2 tomatoes, diced

- 2 tablespoons tomato paste & 1 teaspoon dried thyme

- 1 teaspoon dried oregano & Salt and pepper to taste

- Fresh basil for garnish

Preparation:

1. Preheat the oven to 375°F (190°C).

2. In a large skillet, heat olive oil over medium heat. Add diced eggplant, zucchini, bellpepper, onion, and garlic. Sauté until vegetables are slightly softened. 3. Add diced tomatoes, tomato paste, dried thyme, dried oregano, salt, and pepper to the skillet. Stir to combine.

4. Transfer the vegetable mixture to a baking dish.

5. Cover the baking dish with aluminum foil and bake in the preheated oven for 25-30 minutes, until vegetables are tender.

6. Remove the foil and bake for an additional 10 minutes to allow the top to brown slightly.

7. Garnish with fresh basil before serving.

Nutritional Value (per serving):

- Calories: 200

- Protein: 5g

- Carbohydrates: 40g

- Fat: 3g

Cooking Time: 45 minutes.

5. Vegan Lentil Loaf

Ingredients:

- 1 cup dry green lentils

- 2 cups vegetable broth

- 1 onion, diced

- 2 cloves garlic, minced

- 1 carrot, grated

- 1 celery stalk, diced

- 1/2 cup breadcrumbs

- 2 tablespoons tomato paste

- 1 tablespoon soy sauce

- 1 tablespoon ground flaxseeds mixed with 3 tablespoons water (flax egg)

- 1 teaspoon dried thyme

- 1 teaspoon dried rosemary

- Salt and pepper to taste

Preparation:

1. Preheat the oven to 375°F (190°C).

2. In a pot, combine lentils and vegetable broth. Bring to a boil, then reduce heat and simmer for 20-25 minutes, until lentils are tender and liquid is absorbed.

3. In a skillet, heat olive oil over medium heat. Add diced onion and garlic. Sauté until softened.

4. Add grated carrot, diced celery, cooked lentils, breadcrumbs, tomato paste, soy sauce, flax egg, dried thyme, dried rosemary, salt, and pepper to the skillet. Stir until well combined.

5. Transfer the lentil mixture to a greased loaf pan.

6. Bake in the preheated oven for 40-45 minutes, until the loaf is firm and golden brown on top.

7. Let the lentil loaf cool for a few minutes before slicing and serving.

Nutritional Value (per serving): Calories: 250, Protein: 12g, Carbohydrates: 40g, Fat: 5g

Cooking Time: 60 minutes

Ingredients:

- 1 small butternut squash, peeled and diced

- 1 onion, diced

- 2 cloves garlic, minced

- 1 carrot, diced

- 1 apple, peeled and diced

- 4 cups vegetable broth

- 1 teaspoon curry powder

- 1/2 teaspoon ground ginger

- Salt and pepper to taste

- Coconut cream for garnish

- Fresh parsley for garnish

Preparation:

1. In a large pot, heat olive oil over medium heat. Add diced onion and garlic. Sauté until softened.

2. Add diced butternut squash, carrot, apple, vegetable broth, curry powder, ground ginger, salt, and pepper to the pot. Bring to a boil.

3. Reduce heat and simmer for 20-25 minutes, until the vegetables are tender.

4. Use an immersion blender to blend the soup until smooth. Alternatively, carefully transfer the soup to a blender and blend in batches.

5. Serve hot, garnished with a swirl of coconut cream and fresh parsley.

Nutritional Value (per serving):

- Calories: 200

- Protein: 3g

- Carbohydrates: 45g

- Fat: 2g

Cooking Time: 40 minutes

7. Vegan Cauliflower Alfredo

Ingredients:

- 1 head cauliflower, chopped into florets

- 2 cloves garlic, minced & 2 cups vegetable broth

- 1/2 cup unsweetened almond milk

- 2 tablespoons nutritional yeast

- 1 tablespoon lemon juice & 1 teaspoon Dijon mustard

- Salt and pepper to taste & Cooked pasta of your choice

- Fresh parsley for garnish

Preparation:

1. Steam or boil cauliflower florets until very tender.

2. In a blender, combine steamed cauliflower, minced garlic, vegetable broth, almond milk, nutritional yeast, lemon juice, Dijon mustard, salt, and pepper. Blend until smooth and creamy.

3. Pour the cauliflower Alfredo sauce over cooked pasta of your choice.

4. Garnish with fresh parsley before serving.

Nutritional Value (per serving): Calories: 250, Protein: 10g, Carbohydrates: 40g, Fat: 5g

Cooking Time: 30 minutes

8. Vegan Quinoa Stuffed Bell Peppers

Ingredients:

- 4 bell peppers, halved and seeds removed & 1 cup cooked quinoa

- 1 can (15 oz) black beans, drained and rinsed & 1 cup corn kernels

- 1 cup diced tomatoes & 1 teaspoon chili powder

- 1/2 teaspoon cumin,Salt and pepper to taste & Fresh cilantro for garnish

Preparation:

1. Preheat the oven to 375°F (190°C). Arrange halved bell peppers in a baking dish.

2. In a large bowl, mix together cooked quinoa, black beans, corn kernels, diced tomatoes, chili powder, cumin, salt, and pepper.

3. Spoon the quinoa mixture into each bell pepper half.

4. Cover the baking dish with aluminum foil and bake for 25-30 minutes, until the peppers are tender.

5. Remove the foil and bake for an additional 5 minutes to brown the tops.

6. Garnish with fresh cilantro before serving.

Nutritional Value (per serving, 2 pepper halves): Calories: 350, Protein: 15g, Carbohydrates: 50g, Fat: 5g

Cooking Time: 40 minutes

9. Vegan Lentil Tacos

Ingredients:

- 1 cup dry green lentils &2 cups vegetable broth

- 1 onion, diced & 2 cloves garlic, minced

- 1 tablespoon chili powder & 1 teaspoon ground cumin

- 1/2 teaspoon paprika & Salt and pepper to taste

- Taco shells or tortillas & Sliced avocado

- Shredded lettuce & Diced tomatoes

- Salsa & Fresh cilantro for garnish

Preparation:

1. In a pot, combine lentils and vegetable broth. Bring to a boil, then reduce heat and simmer for 20-25 minutes, until lentils are tender.

2. In a skillet, heat olive oil over medium heat. Add diced onion and garlic. Sauté until softened.

3. Add cooked lentils, chili powder, ground cumin, paprika, salt, and pepper to the skillet. Cook for another 5 minutes.

4. Serve the lentil mixture in taco shells or tortillas.

5. Top with sliced avocado, shredded lettuce, diced tomatoes, salsa, and fresh cilantro

   for garnish.

6. Serve immediately.

Nutritional Value (per   serving, 2 tacos): Calories: 350, Protein: 12g, Carbohydrates: 45g, Fat: 10g   **Cooking Time: 30 minutes**

10. Vegan Mushroom Risotto

Ingredients:

- 1 cup Arborio rice & 4 cups vegetable broth

- 1 onion, diced & 2 cloves garlic, minced

- 8 oz mushrooms, sliced & 1/2 cup dry white wine (optional)

- 2 tablespoons nutritional yeast & 2 tablespoons vegan butter

- Salt and pepper to taste & Fresh parsley for garnish

Preparation:

1. In a saucepan, heat vegetable broth over medium heat and keep it simmering.

2. In a separate large skillet, melt vegan butter over medium heat. Add diced onion and minced garlic. Sauté until softened.

3. Add Arborio rice to the skillet and stir to coat with butter.

4. If using, pour in dry white wine and cook until absorbed.

5. Begin adding the simmering vegetable broth, one ladleful at a time, stirring frequently and allowing each addition to be absorbed before adding more. Continue until the rice is creamy and cooked through (about 20-25 minutes).

6. In the last few minutes of cooking, stir in sliced mushrooms and nutritional yeast. Cook until the mushrooms are tender.

7. Season with salt and pepper to taste.

8. Serve hot, garnished with fresh parsley.

Nutritional Value (per serving):

- Calories: 350

- Protein: 8g

- Carbohydrates: 60g

- Fat: 5g

Cooking Time: 35 minutes

11. Vegan Lentil Bolognese

Ingredients:

- 1 cup dry green lentils & 2 cups vegetable broth

- 1 onion, diced & 2 cloves garlic, minced

- 1 carrot, grated & 1 celery stalk, diced

- 1 can (14 oz) crushed tomatoes & 2 tablespoons tomato paste

- 1 teaspoon dried oregano, 1 teaspoon dried basil & Salt and pepper to taste

- Cooked pasta of your choice and Fresh basil for garnish

Preparation:

1. In a pot, combine lentils and vegetable broth. Bring to a boil, then reduce heat and simmer for 20-25 minutes, until lentils are tender and liquid is absorbed.

2. In a skillet, heat olive oil over medium heat. Add diced onion, garlic, grated carrot, and diced celery. Sauté until softened.

3. Add crushed tomatoes, tomato paste, dried oregano, dried basil, cooked lentils,

salt, and pepper to the skillet. Cook for another 10 minutes.

4. Serve the lentil Bolognese sauce over cooked pasta of your choice.

5. Garnish with fresh basil before serving.

Nutritional Value (per serving):

- Calories: 300

- Protein: 12g

- Carbohydrates: 50g

- Fat: 3g

Cooking Time: 35 minutes

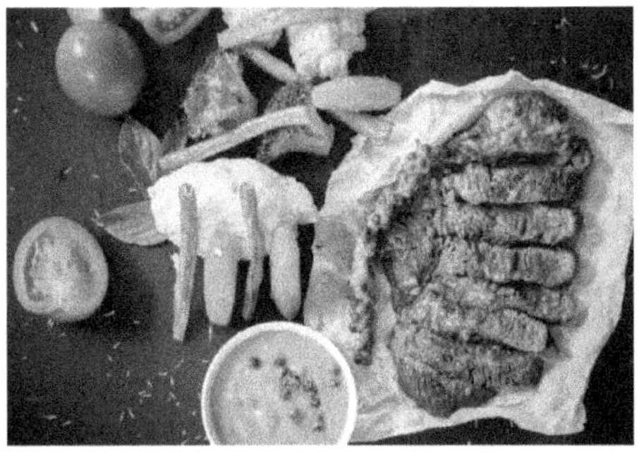

12. Vegan Thai Peanut Noodles

Ingredients:

- 8 oz whole wheat spaghetti or rice noodles

- 1/4 cup peanut butter & 2 tablespoons soy sauce

- 1 tablespoon maple syrup & 1 tablespoon lime juice

- 1 clove garlic, minced & 1 teaspoon grated ginger

- 1/4 cup water & 1 tablespoon sesame oil

- 1 red bell pepper,

- thinly sliced

- 1 carrot, julienned

- 1 cup broccoli florets

- 1/4 cup chopped

- peanuts for garnish

- Fresh cilantro for garnish

Preparation:

1. Cook noodles according to package instructions. Drain and set aside.

2. In a small bowl, whisk together peanut butter, soy sauce, maple syrup, lime juice, minced garlic, grated ginger, and water to make the peanut sauce. Set aside.

3. In a large skillet or wok, heat sesame oil over medium-high heat. Add sliced bell pepper, julienned carrot, and broccoli florets. Stir-fry for 5-7 minutes, until vegetables are tender-crisp.

4. Add cooked noodles to the skillet, then pour the peanut sauce over the noodles and vegetables. Toss until everything is well coated.

5. Serve hot, garnished with chopped peanuts and fresh cilantro.

Nutritional Value (per serving): Calories: 400

Protein: 15gCarbohydrates: 50g, Fat: 18g

Cooking Time: 20 minutes

13. Vegan Sweet Potato & Black Bean Chili

Ingredients:

- 2 sweet potatoes, peeled and diced

- 1 onion, diced

- 2 cloves garlic, minced

- 1 red bell pepper, diced

- 1 can (15 oz) black beans, drained and rinsed

- 1 can (14 oz) diced tomatoes

- 2 cups vegetable broth

- 1 tablespoon chili powder

- 1 teaspoon cumin

- 1/2 teaspoon smoked paprika

- Salt and pepper to taste

- Fresh cilantro for garnish

Preparation:

1. In a large pot, heat olive oil over medium heat. Add diced onion, minced garlic, and diced bell pepper. Sauté until softened.

2. Add diced sweet potatoes, black beans, diced tomatoes, vegetable broth, chili powder, cumin, smoked paprika, salt, and pepper to the pot. Stir to combine.

3. Bring the chili to a simmer, then reduce heat and cook for 20-25 minutes, until sweet potatoes are tender.

4. Serve hot, garnished with fresh cilantro.

Nutritional Value (per serving):

- Calories: 300

- Protein: 10g

- Carbohydrates: 50g

- Fat: 5g

Cooking Time: 35 minutes

14. Vegan Mediterranean Stuffed Portobello Mushrooms

Ingredients:

- 4 large portobello mushrooms, stems removed & 1 cup cooked quinoa

- 1/2 cup diced tomatoes & 1/4 cup sliced Kalamata olives

- 1/4 cup chopped fresh parsley & 2 cloves garlic, minced

- 2 tablespoons olive oil & 2 tablespoons balsamic vinegar

- Salt and pepper to taste

Preparation:

1. Preheat the oven to 375°F (190°C). Place portobello mushrooms on a baking sheet lined with parchment paper.

2. In a bowl, mix together cooked quinoa,

   diced tomatoes, sliced Kalamata olives, chopped fresh parsley, minced garlic, olive oil, balsamic vinegar, salt, and pepper. 3. Spoon the quinoa mixture into the cavity of each portobello mushroom, pressing down gently to pack the filling.

4. Bake in the preheated oven for 20-25 minutes, until the mushrooms are tender and the filling is heated through.

5. Serve hot, garnished with additional parsley if desired.

Nutritional Value (per serving):

- Calories: 250

- Protein: 8g

- Carbohydrates: 35g

- Fat: 10g

Cooking Time: 30 minutes

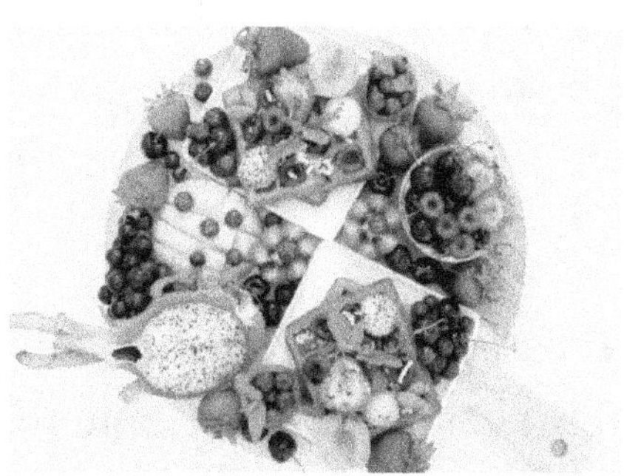

15. Vegan Lentil & Vegetable Soup

Ingredients:

- 1 cup dry green lentils & 4 cups vegetable broth

- 1 onion, diced & 2 cloves garlic, minced

- 2 carrots, diced & 2 celery stalks, diced

- 1 zucchini, diced & 1 can (14 oz) diced tomatoes

- 1 teaspoon dried thyme & 1 teaspoon dried rosemary

- Salt and pepper to taste & Fresh parsley for garnish

Preparation:

1. In a pot, combine lentils and vegetable broth. Bring to a boil, then reduce heat and simmer for 20-25 minutes, until lentils are tender.

2. In a separate large pot, heat olive oil over medium heat. Add diced onion and minced garlic. Sauté until softened.

3. Add diced carrots, celery, and zucchini to the pot. Sauté for another 5 minutes.

4. Pour in diced tomatoes (with their juices) and cooked lentils with broth.

5. Stir in dried thyme, dried rosemary, salt, and pepper.

6. Simmer the soup for 15-20 minutes, until the vegetables are tender and flavors are well combined.

7. Adjust seasoning if needed.

8. Serve hot, garnished with fresh parsley.

Nutritional Value (per serving):

- Calories: 300

- Protein: 15g

- Carbohydrates: 50g

- Fat: 5g

Cooking Time: 45 minutes

1. Chia Seed Pudding

Ingredients:

- 3 tablespoons chia seeds

- 1 cup almond milk

- 1 tablespoon maple syrup

- Fresh berries for topping

Preparation:

1. In a bowl, mix chia seeds, almond milk, and maple syrup.

2. Let it sit in the refrigerator for at least 2 hours or overnight until thickened.

3. Serve chilled, topped with fresh berries.

Nutritional Value (per serving): Calories: 150, Protein: 4g, Carbohydrates: 15g, Fat: 8g

Ingredients:

- 1 cup cooked chickpeas

- 2 tablespoons tahini

- 1 clove garlic, minced

- Juice of 1 lemon

- Salt and pepper to taste

- Carrot sticks, cucumber slices, and bell pepper strips for dipping

Preparation:

1. In a food processor, blend chickpeas, tahini, minced garlic, lemon juice, salt, and pepper until smooth.

2. Serve with veggie sticks for dipping.

Nutritional Value (per serving):

Calories: 150 Protein: 5g, Carbohydrates: 20g, Fat: 7g

3. Vegan Yogurt Parfait

Ingredients:

- 1 cup dairy-free yogurt

- 1/4 cup granola

- Fresh berries

- Drizzle of maple syrup (optional)

Preparation:

1. In a glass, layer dairy-free yogurt, granola, and fresh berries.

2. Drizzle with maple syrup if desired.

3. Serve immediately.

Nutritional Value (per serving):

Calories: 200, Protein: 8g, Carbohydrates: 30g, Fat: 5g

4. Avocado Toast

Ingredients:

- 1 ripe avocado

- 2 slices whole grain bread

- Salt, pepper, and red pepper flakes to taste

- Optional toppings: sliced tomato, sprouts, or hemp seeds

Preparation:

1. Toast the bread slices until golden brown.

2. Mash the ripe avocado and spread it evenly on the toast.

3. Season with salt, pepper, and red pepper flakes.

4. Add optional toppings if desired.

5. Serve immediately.

Nutritional Value (per serving):

Calories: 250 Protein: 6g, Carbohydrates: 30g, Fat: 12g

5. Trail Mix

Ingredients:

- 1/2 cup almonds

- 1/2 cup walnuts

- 1/4 cup pumpkin seeds

- 1/4 cup dried cranberries

- 1/4 cup dark chocolate chips

Preparation:

1. Mix all ingredients together in a bowl.

2. Store in an airtight container for snacking.

Nutritional Value (per serving):

Calories: 200, Protein: 5g, Carbohydrates: 15g, Fat: 15g

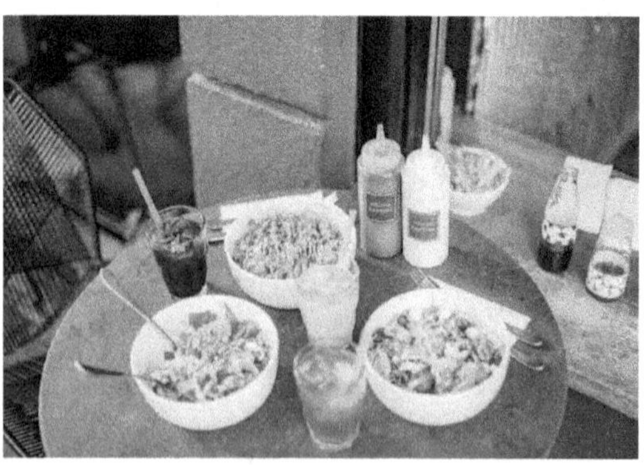

6. Veggie Sushi Rolls

Ingredients:

- Nori sheets

- Cooked quinoa or sushi rice

- Thinly sliced cucumber, avocado, and bell peppers

- Soy sauce or tamari for dipping

Preparation:

1. Place a nori sheet on a bamboo sushi mat.

2. Spread cooked quinoa or sushi rice evenly over the nori sheet.

3. Add thinly sliced cucumber, avocado, and bell peppers on top of the rice.

4. Roll tightly using the sushi mat.

5. Slice into bite-sized pieces.

6. Serve with soy sauce or tamari for dipping.

Nutritional Value (per serving): Calories: 180 Protein: 5g, Carbohydrates: 30g, Fat: 5g

7. Edamame

Ingredients:

- 1 cup frozen edamame

- Salt to taste Preparation:

1. Boil or steam frozen edamame according to package instructions.

2. Season with salt to taste.

3. Serve warm or chilled.

Nutritional Value (per serving):

- Calories: 100

- Protein: 8g

- Carbohydrates: 9g

- Fat: 4g

Ingredients:

- Medjool dates, pitted

- Almond or peanut butter

- Optional toppings: chopped nuts, shredded coconut, or dark chocolate chips

Preparation:

1. Fill each pitted date with almond or peanut butter.

2. Sprinkle with optional toppings if desired.

3. Serve immediately.

Nutritional Value (per serving):

- Calories: 120

- Protein: 2g

- Carbohydrates: 25g

- Fat: 3g

9. Crispy Kale Chips

Ingredients:

- 1 bunch kale, washed and dried

- 1 tablespoon olive oil

- Salt and nutritional yeast to taste

Preparation:

1. Preheat the oven to 350°F (175°C).

2. Remove the stems from the kale leaves and tear them into bite-sized pieces.

3. In a bowl, toss kale pieces with olive oil, salt, and nutritional yeast.

4. Spread kale pieces in a single layer on a baking sheet.

5. Bake for 10-15 minutes until crispy.

6. Let cool before serving.

Nutritional Value (per serving):

Calories: 100, Protein: 5g, Carbohydrates: 10g, Fat: 6g

Ingredients:

- Assorted fresh fruits (such as berries, oranges, kiwi, and grapes)

- Fresh mint leaves for garnish

Preparation:

1. Wash and chop assorted fruits into bite-sized pieces.

2. Mix together in a bowl.

3. Garnish with fresh mint leaves.

4. Serve immediately

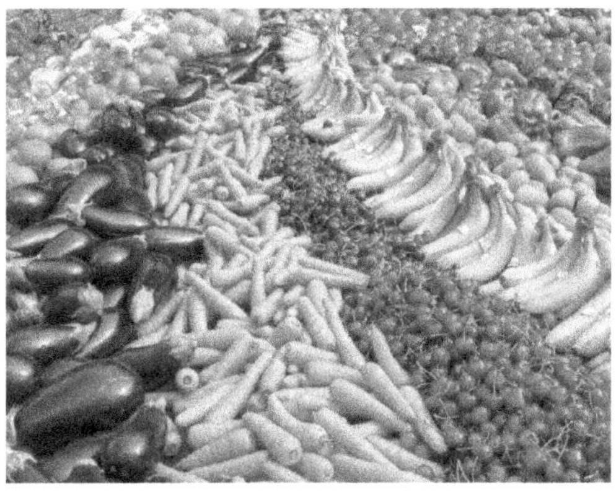

11. Roasted Chickpeas

Ingredients:

- 1 can (15 oz) chickpeas, drained and rinsed
- 1 tablespoon olive oil
- 1 teaspoon paprika
- 1/2 teaspoon cumin & Salt to taste

Preparation:

1. Preheat the oven to 400°F (200°C).

2. Pat dry the chickpeas using a kitchen towel to remove excess moisture.

3. In a bowl, toss chickpeas with olive oil, paprika, cumin, and salt until evenly coated.

4. Spread chickpeas in a single layer on a baking sheet.

5. Roast for 25-30 minutes, stirring occasionally, until crispy.

6. Let cool before serving.

   Nutritional Value (per serving): Calories: 150, Protein: 6g, Carbohydrates: 20g, Fat: 5g

Ingredients:

- 1 ripe banana, mashed & 1 cup rolled oats

- 1/4 cup almond butter & 2 tablespoons maple syrup

- 1/4 cup chopped nuts or seeds

Preparation:

1. In a bowl, combine mashed banana, rolled oats, almond butter, maple syrup, and chopped nuts or seeds.

2. Mix until well combined.

3. Roll the mixture into small balls using your hands.

4. Place the balls on a baking sheet lined with parchment paper.

5. Refrigerate for at least 30 minutes before serving.

Nutritional Value (per serving): Calories: 120, Protein: 4g, Carbohydrates: 15g, Fat: 6g

13. Cucumber Avocado Rolls

Ingredients:

- 1 cucumber & 1 avocado

- Juice of 1/2 lemon & Salt and pepper to taste

- Optional fillings: shredded carrots, sprouts, or hummus

Preparation:

1. Slice the cucumber lengthwise into thin strips using a vegetable peeler or mandoline.

2. In a bowl, mash the avocado with lemon juice, salt, and pepper.

3. Spread a thin layer of mashed avocado onto each cucumber strip.

4. Add optional fillings if desired.

5. Roll up the cucumber strips and secure with toothpicks.

6. Serve immediately.

Nutritional Value (per serving): Calories: 80, Protein: 2g, Carbohydrates: 6g, Fat: 6g

14. Coconut Yogurt with Berries

Ingredients:

- 1 cup dairy-free coconut yogurt

- 1/2 cup mixed berries (such as strawberries, blueberries, and raspberries)

- 1 tablespoon shredded coconut

- Optional: drizzle of honey or maple syrup

Preparation:

1. In a bowl, spoon coconut yogurt.

2. Top with mixed berries and shredded coconut.

3. Drizzle with honey or maple syrup if desired.

4. Serve immediately.

Nutritional Value (per serving):

- Calories: 150, Protein: 3g, Carbohydrates: 20g, Fat: 7g

15. Apple Sandwiches with Almond Butter

Ingredients:

- 1 apple, cored and sliced into rounds

- Almond butter

- Optional toppings: sliced bananas, raisins, or cinnamon

Preparation:

1. Spread almond butter on one apple slice.

2. Top with another apple slice to create a sandwich.

3. Add optional toppings if desired.

4. Repeat to make more sandwiches.

5. Serve immediately or pack for on-the-go snacking.

Nutritional Value (per serving):

Calories: 150, Protein: 3g, Carbohydrates: 20g, Fat: 7g

1. Chia Seed Pudding

Ingredients:

- 3 tablespoons chia seeds

- 1 cup almond milk

- 1 tablespoon maple syrup

- Fresh berries for topping

Preparation:

1. In a bowl, mix chia seeds, almond milk, and maple syrup.

2. Let it sit in the refrigerator for at least 2 hours or overnight until thickened.

3. Serve chilled, topped with fresh berries.

Nutritional Value (per serving):

Calories: 150, Protein: 4g, Carbohydrates: 15g, Fat: 8g

2. Hummus and Veggie Sticks

Ingredients:

- 1 cup cooked chickpeas

- 2 tablespoons tahini

- 1 clove garlic, minced

- Juice of 1 lemon

- Salt and pepper to taste

- Carrot sticks, cucumber slices, and bell pepper strips for dipping

Preparation:

1. In a food processor, blend chickpeas, tahini, minced garlic, lemon juice, salt, and pepper until smooth.

2. Serve with veggie sticks for dipping.

Nutritional Value (per serving):

Calories: 150, Protein: 5g, Carbohydrates: 20g, Fat: 7g

Ingredients:

- 1 cup dairy-free yogurt

- 1/4 cup granola

- Fresh berries

- Drizzle of maple syrup (optional)

Preparation:

1. In a glass, layer dairy-free yogurt, granola, and fresh berries.

2. Drizzle with maple syrup if desired.

3. Serve immediately.

Nutritional Value (per serving):

- Calories: 200

- Protein: 8g

- Carbohydrates: 30g

- Fat: 5g

4. Avocado Toast

Ingredients:

- 1 ripe avocado

- 2 slices whole grain bread

- Salt, pepper, and red pepper flakes to taste

- Optional toppings: sliced tomato, sprouts, or hemp seeds

Preparation:

1. Toast the bread slices until golden brown.

2. Mash the ripe avocado and spread it evenly on the toast.

3. Season with salt, pepper, and red pepper flakes.

4. Add optional toppings if desired.

5. Serve immediately.

Nutritional Value (per serving):

Calories: 250, Protein: 6g, Carbohydrates: 30g, Fat: 12g

5. Trail Mix

Ingredients:

- 1/2 cup almonds

- 1/2 cup walnuts

- 1/4 cup pumpkin seeds

- 1/4 cup dried cranberries

- 1/4 cup dark chocolate chips

Preparation:

1. Mix all ingredients together in a bowl.

2. Store in an airtight container for snacking.

Nutritional Value (per serving):

- Calories: 200

- Protein: 5g

- Carbohydrates: 15g

- Fat: 15g

6. Veggie Sushi Rolls

Ingredients:

- Nori sheets

- Cooked quinoa or sushi rice

- Thinly sliced cucumber, avocado, and bell peppers

- Soy sauce or tamari for dipping

Preparation:

1. Place a nori sheet on a bamboo sushi mat.

2. Spread cooked quinoa or sushi rice evenly over the nori sheet.

3. Add thinly sliced cucumber, avocado, and bell peppers on top of the rice.

4. Roll tightly using the sushi mat.

5. Slice into bite-sized pieces.

6. Serve with soy sauce or tamari for dipping.

Nutritional Value (per serving): Calories: 180, Protein: 5g, Carbohydrates: 30g, Fat: 5g

7. Edamame

Ingredients:

- 1 cup frozen edamame
- Salt to taste

Preparation:

1. Boil or steam frozen edamame according to package instructions.
2. Season with salt to taste.
3. Serve warm or chilled.

Nutritional Value (per serving):

- Calories: 100
- Protein: 8g
- Carbohydrates: 9g
- Fat: 4g

8. Stuffed Dates

Ingredients:

- Medjool dates, pitted

- Almond or peanut butter

- Optional toppings: chopped nuts, shredded coconut, or dark chocolate chips

Preparation:

1. Fill each pitted date with almond or peanut butter.

2. Sprinkle with optional toppings if desired.

3. Serve immediately.

Nutritional Value (per serving):

- Calories: 120

- Protein: 2g

- Carbohydrates: 25g

- Fat: 3g

9. Crispy Kale Chips

Ingredients:

- 1 bunch kale, washed and dried

- 1 tablespoon olive oil

- Salt and nutritional yeast to taste

Preparation:

1. Preheat the oven to 350°F (175°C).

2. Remove the stems from the kale leaves and tear them into bite-sized pieces.

3. In a bowl, toss kale pieces with olive oil, salt, and nutritional yeast.

4. Spread kale pieces in a single layer on a baking sheet.

5. Bake for 10-15 minutes until crispy.

6. Let cool before serving

Nutritional Value (per serving):

Calories: 100, Protein: 5g, Carbohydrates: 10g, Fat: 6g

Ingredients:

- Assorted fresh fruits (such as berries, oranges, kiwi, and grapes)

- Fresh mint leaves for garnish

Preparation:

1. Wash and chop assorted fruits into bite-sized pieces.

2. Mix together in a bowl.

3. Garnish with fresh mint leaves.

4. Serve immediately

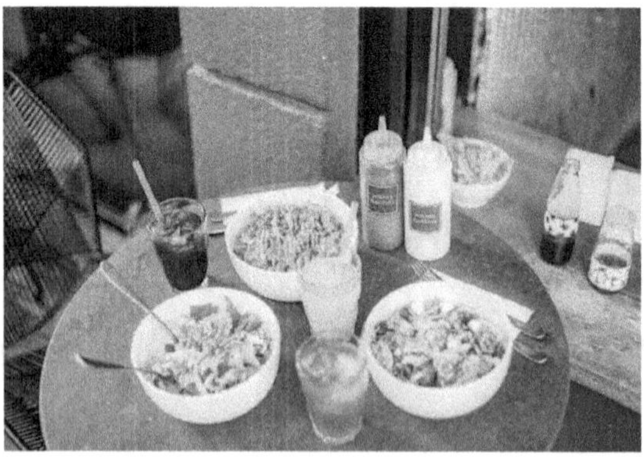

Ingredients:

- 1 can (15 oz) chickpeas, drained and rinsed
- 1 tablespoon olive oil
- 1 teaspoon paprika
- 1/2 teaspoon cumin
- Salt to taste

Preparation:

1. Preheat the oven to 400°F (200°C).
2. Pat dry the chickpeas using a kitchen towel to remove excess moisture.
3. In a bowl, toss chickpeas with olive oil, paprika, cumin, and salt until evenly coated.
4. Spread chickpeas in a single layer on a baking sheet.
5. Roast for 25-30 minutes, stirring occasionally, until crispy.
6. Let cool before serving.

Nutritional Value (per serving): Calories: 150, Protein: 6g, Carbohydrates: 20g, Fat: 5g

12. Banana-Oat Energy Bites

Ingredients:

- 1 ripe banana, mashed &1 cup rolled oats

- 1/4 cup almond butter

- 2 tablespoons maple syrup

- 1/4 cup chopped nuts or seeds

Preparation:

1. In a bowl, combine mashed banana, rolled oats, almond butter, maple syrup, and chopped nuts or seeds.

2. Mix until well combined.

3. Roll the mixture into small balls using your hands.

4. Place the balls on a baking sheet lined with parchment paper.

5. Refrigerate for at least 30 minutes before serving.

Nutritional Value (per serving):

Calories: 120, Protein: 4g, Carbohydrates: 15g, Fat: 6g

13. Cucumber Avocado Rolls

Ingredients:

- 1 cucumber & 1 avocado

- Juice of 1/2 lemon

- Salt and pepper to taste

- Optional fillings: shredded carrots, sprouts, or hummus

Preparation:

1. Slice the cucumber lengthwise into thin strips using a vegetable peeler or mandoline.

2. In a bowl, mash the avocado with lemon juice, salt, and pepper.

3. Spread a thin layer of mashed avocado onto each cucumber strip.

4. Add optional fillings if desired.

5. Roll up the cucumber strips and secure with toothpicks.

6. Serve immediately.

Nutritional Value (per serving): Calories: 80, Protein: 2g, Carbohydrates: 6g, Fat: 6g

14. Coconut Yogurt with Berries

Ingredients:

- 1 cup dairy-free coconut yogurt

- 1/2 cup mixed berries (such as strawberries, blueberries, and raspberries)

- 1 tablespoon shredded coconut

- Optional: drizzle of honey or maple syrup

Preparation:

1. In a bowl, spoon coconut yogurt.

2. Top with mixed berries and shredded coconut.

3. Drizzle with honey or maple syrup if desired and serve immediately.

Nutritional Value (per serving): Calories: 150

Protein: 3g, Carbohydrates: 20g, Fat: 7g

15. Apple Sandwiches with Almond Butter

Ingredients:

- 1 apple, cored and sliced into rounds & Almond butter

- Optional toppings: sliced bananas, raisins, or cinnamon

Preparation:

1. Spread almond butter on one apple slice.

2. Top with another apple slice to create a sandwich.

3. Add optional toppings if desired.

4. Repeat to make more sandwiches.

5. Serve immediately or pack for on-the-go snacking.

Nutritional Value (per serving):

- Calories: 150

- Protein: 3g

- Carbohydrates: 20g

- Fat: 7g

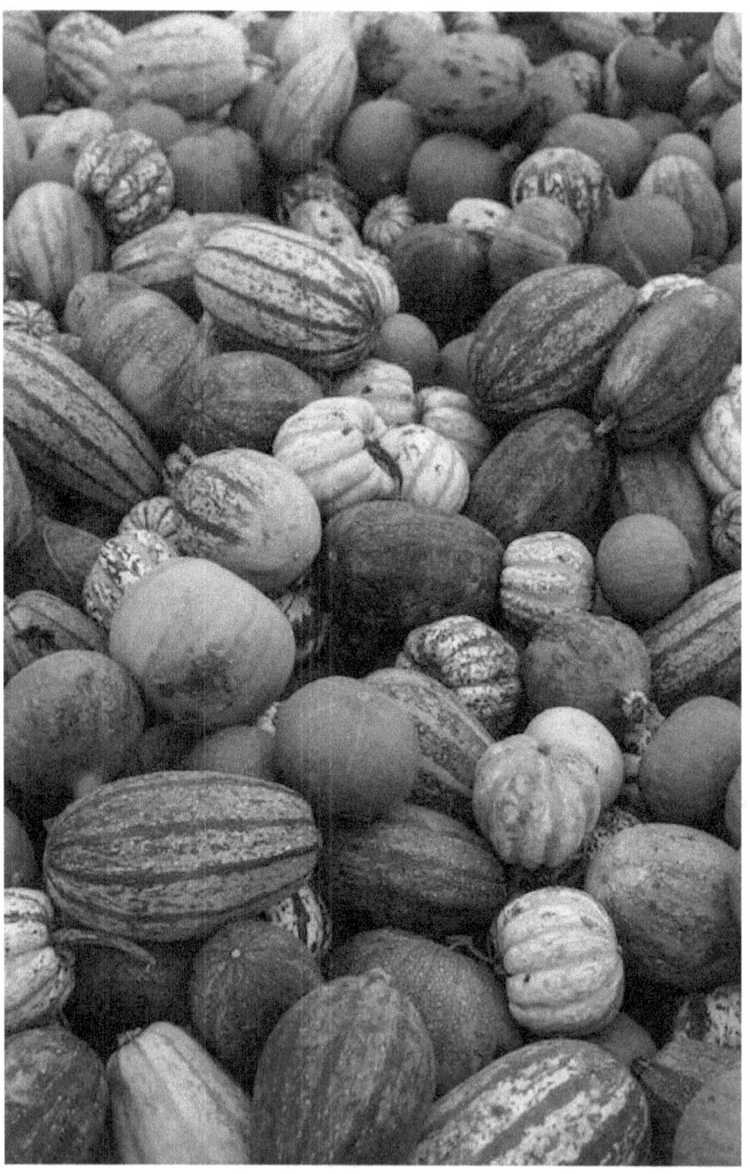

In conclusion, the Menopause Vegan Diet Cookbook presents a comprehensive array of delicious, nutritious, and inflammation-fighting recipes tailored specifically for individuals navigating the challenges of menopause. Through a carefully curated selection of breakfasts, lunches, dinners, snacks, and desserts, this cookbook offers flavorful options to support hormonal balance, alleviate symptoms, and promote overall health and well-being during this transformative stage of life. By embracing a plant-based diet rich in whole foods, antioxidants, and essential nutrients, individuals can empower themselves to naturally combat menopausal symptoms and optimize their health.

Embarking on this journey towards a menopause-friendly vegan diet isn't just about nourishing the body; it's about embracing a lifestyle that honors both physical and emotional wellness. Each recipe in this cookbook is not only a culinary delight but also a step towards self-care and empowerment. With dedication and commitment, readers can discover the transformative power of food and unlock the potential for a vibrant, fulfilling life beyond menopause.

Let this cookbook be your guide on the path to better health and vitality. Embrace the journey, savor the flavors, and nourish your body with the wholesome goodness of plant-based nutrition. Your health and well-being are worth every flavorful bite.

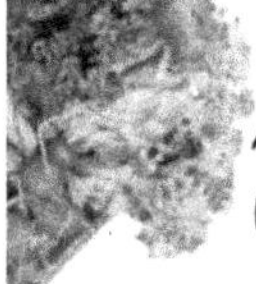

WEEKIY MEAL PLANNER

MONDAY	BREAKFAST	
	LUNCH	
	DINNER	
TUESDAY	BREAKFAST	
	LUNCH	
	DINNER	
WEDNESDAY	BREAKFAST	
	LUNCH	
	DINNER	
THURSDAY	BREAKFAST	
	LUNCH	
	DINNER	
FRIDAY	BREAKFAST	
	LUNCH	
	DINNER	
SARTURDAY	BREAKFAST	
	LUNCH	
	DINNER	
SUNDAY	BREAKFAST	
	LUNCH	
	DINNER	

GROCERY LIST

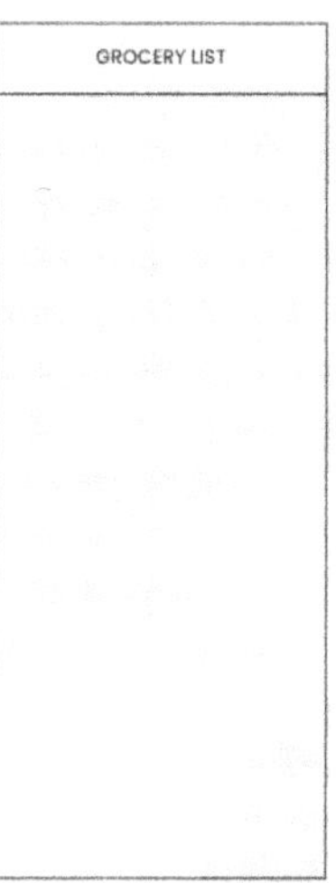

SNACKS

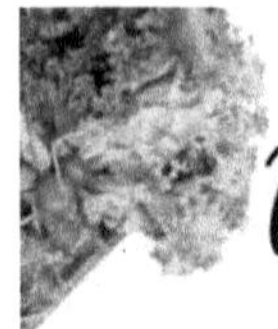

WEEKIY MEAL PLANNER

MONDAY	BREAKFAST	
	LUNCH	
	DINNER	
TUESDAY	BREAKFAST	
	LUNCH	
	DINNER	
WEDNESDAY	BREAKFAST	
	LUNCH	
	DINNER	
THURSDAY	BREAKFAST	
	LUNCH	
	DINNER	
FRIDAY	BREAKFAST	
	LUNCH	
	DINNER	
SARTURDAY	BREAKFAST	
	LUNCH	
	DINNER	
SUNDAY	BREAKFAST	
	LUNCH	
	DINNER	

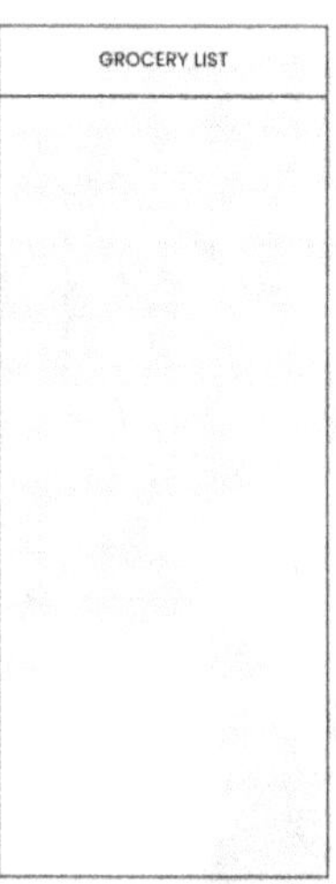

GROCERY LIST

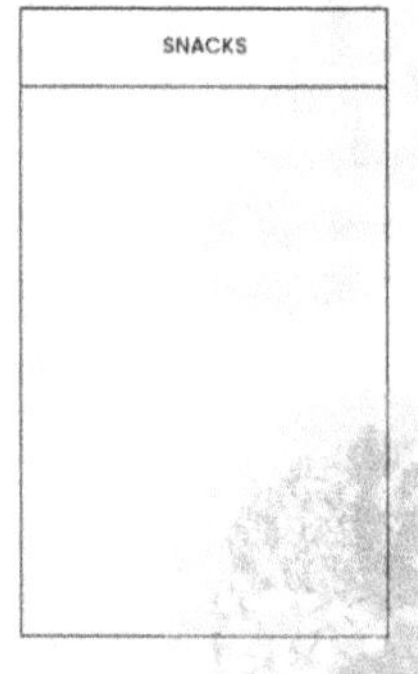

SNACKS

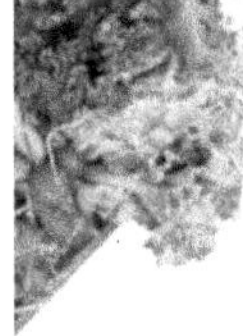

WEEKLY MEAL PLANNER

MONDAY	BREAKFAST	
	LUNCH	
	DINNER	
TUESDAY	BREAKFAST	
	LUNCH	
	DINNER	
WEDNESDAY	BREAKFAST	
	LUNCH	
	DINNER	
THURSDAY	BREAKFAST	
	LUNCH	
	DINNER	
FRIDAY	BREAKFAST	
	LUNCH	
	DINNER	
SARTURDAY	BREAKFAST	
	LUNCH	
	DINNER	
SUNDAY	BREAKFAST	
	LUNCH	
	DINNER	

GROCERY LIST

SNACKS

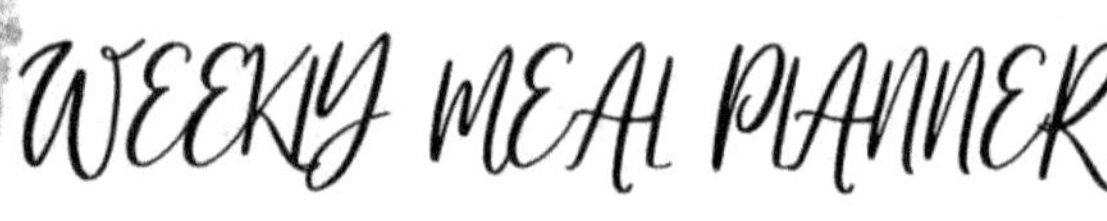

MONDAY	BREAKFAST	
	LUNCH	
	DINNER	
TUESDAY	BREAKFAST	
	LUNCH	
	DINNER	
WEDNESDAY	BREAKFAST	
	LUNCH	
	DINNER	
THURSDAY	BREAKFAST	
	LUNCH	
	DINNER	
FRIDAY	BREAKFAST	
	LUNCH	
	DINNER	
SARTURDAY	BREAKFAST	
	LUNCH	
	DINNER	
SUNDAY	BREAKFAST	
	LUNCH	
	DINNER	

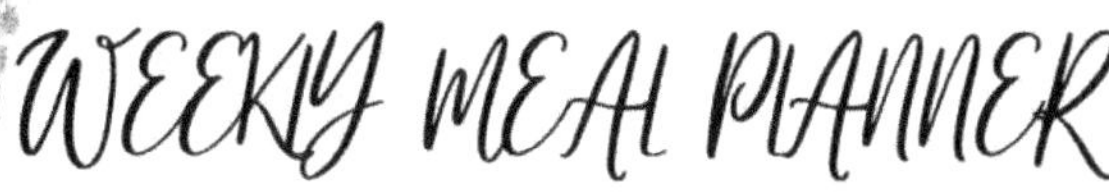

WEEKLY MEAL PLANNER

MONDAY	BREAKFAST	
	LUNCH	
	DINNER	
TUESDAY	BREAKFAST	
	LUNCH	
	DINNER	
WEDNESDAY	BREAKFAST	
	LUNCH	
	DINNER	
THURSDAY	BREAKFAST	
	LUNCH	
	DINNER	
FRIDAY	BREAKFAST	
	LUNCH	
	DINNER	
SARTURDAY	BREAKFAST	
	LUNCH	
	DINNER	
SUNDAY	BREAKFAST	
	LUNCH	
	DINNER	

GROCERY LIST

SNACKS

WEEKLY MEAL PLANNER

MONDAY	BREAKFAST	
	LUNCH	
	DINNER	
TUESDAY	BREAKFAST	
	LUNCH	
	DINNER	
WEDNESDAY	BREAKFAST	
	LUNCH	
	DINNER	
THURSDAY	BREAKFAST	
	LUNCH	
	DINNER	
FRIDAY	BREAKFAST	
	LUNCH	
	DINNER	
SARTURDAY	BREAKFAST	
	LUNCH	
	DINNER	
SUNDAY	BREAKFAST	
	LUNCH	
	DINNER	

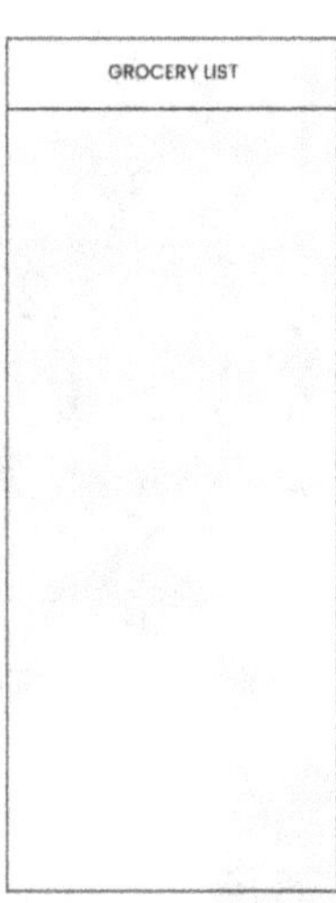

GROCERY LIST

SNACKS

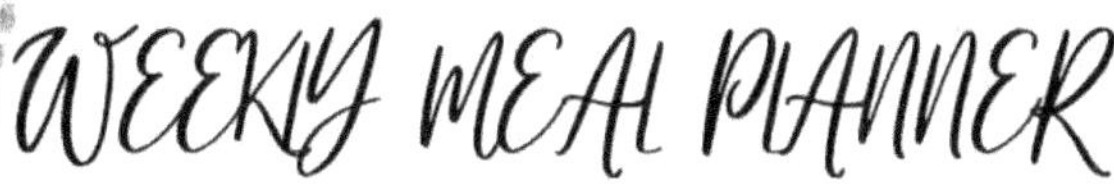

WEEKLY MEAL PLANNER

MONDAY	BREAKFAST	
	LUNCH	
	DINNER	

TUESDAY	BREAKFAST	
	LUNCH	
	DINNER	

WEDNESDAY	BREAKFAST	
	LUNCH	
	DINNER	

THURSDAY	BREAKFAST	
	LUNCH	
	DINNER	

FRIDAY	BREAKFAST	
	LUNCH	
	DINNER	

SARTURDAY	BREAKFAST	
	LUNCH	
	DINNER	

SUNDAY	BREAKFAST	
	LUNCH	
	DINNER	

GROCERY LIST

SNACKS

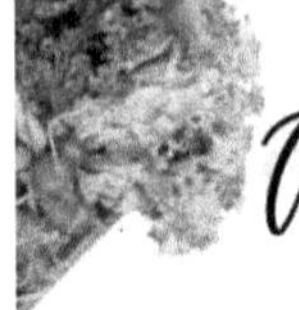

WEEKLY MEAL PLANNER

MONDAY	BREAKFAST	
	LUNCH	
	DINNER	
TUESDAY	BREAKFAST	
	LUNCH	
	DINNER	
WEDNESDAY	BREAKFAST	
	LUNCH	
	DINNER	
THURSDAY	BREAKFAST	
	LUNCH	
	DINNER	
FRIDAY	BREAKFAST	
	LUNCH	
	DINNER	
SARTURDAY	BREAKFAST	
	LUNCH	
	DINNER	
SUNDAY	BREAKFAST	
	LUNCH	
	DINNER	

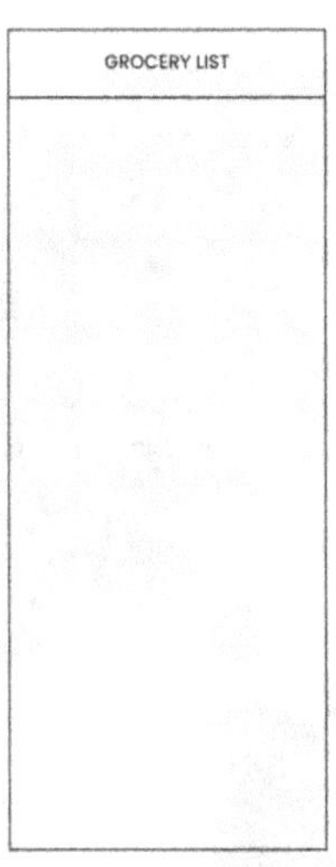

GROCERY LIST

SNACKS

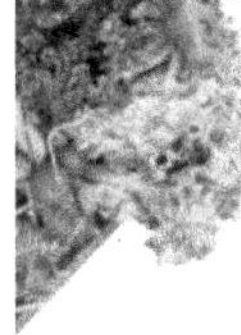

WEEKIY MEAI PIANNER

MONDAY	BREAKFAST	
	LUNCH	
	DINNER	
TUESDAY	BREAKFAST	
	LUNCH	
	DINNER	
WEDNESDAY	BREAKFAST	
	LUNCH	
	DINNER	
THURSDAY	BREAKFAST	
	LUNCH	
	DINNER	
FRIDAY	BREAKFAST	
	LUNCH	
	DINNER	
SARTURDAY	BREAKFAST	
	LUNCH	
	DINNER	
SUNDAY	BREAKFAST	
	LUNCH	
	DINNER	

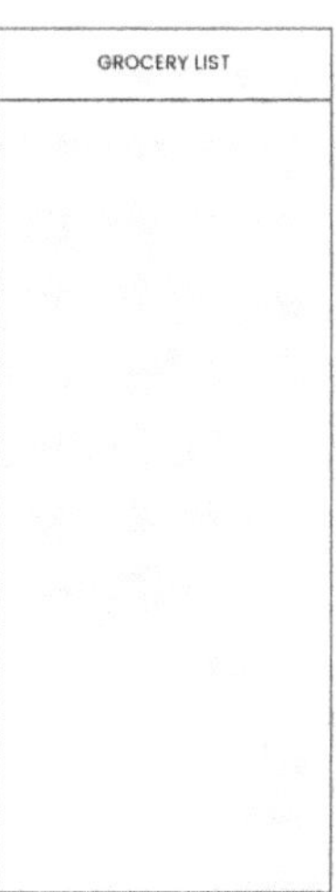

GROCERY LIST

SNACKS

WEEKLY MEAL PLANNER

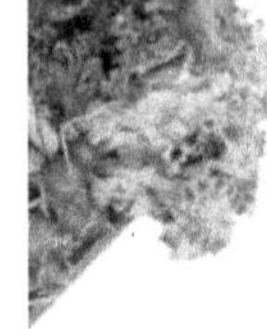

			GROCERY LIST
MONDAY	BREAKFAST		
	LUNCH		
	DINNER		
TUESDAY	BREAKFAST		
	LUNCH		
	DINNER		
WEDNESDAY	BREAKFAST		
	LUNCH		
	DINNER		
THURSDAY	BREAKFAST		
	LUNCH		
	DINNER		
FRIDAY	BREAKFAST		SNACKS
	LUNCH		
	DINNER		
SARTURDAY	BREAKFAST		
	LUNCH		
	DINNER		
SUNDAY	BREAKFAST		
	LUNCH		
	DINNER		

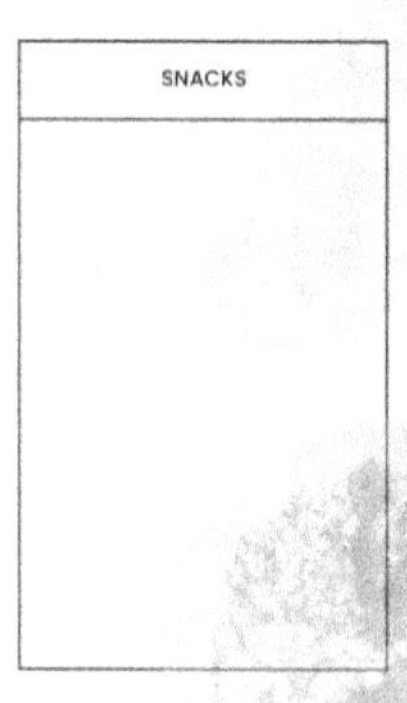

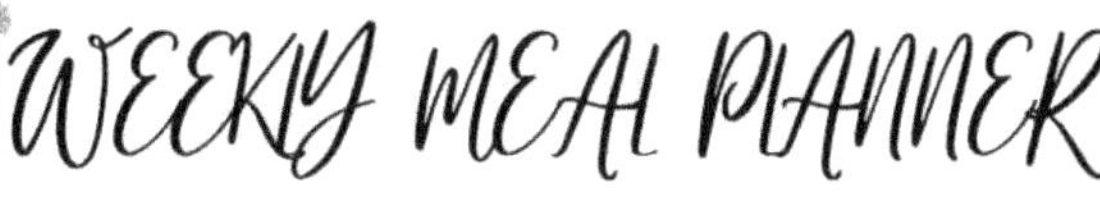

			GROCERY LIST
MONDAY	BREAKFAST		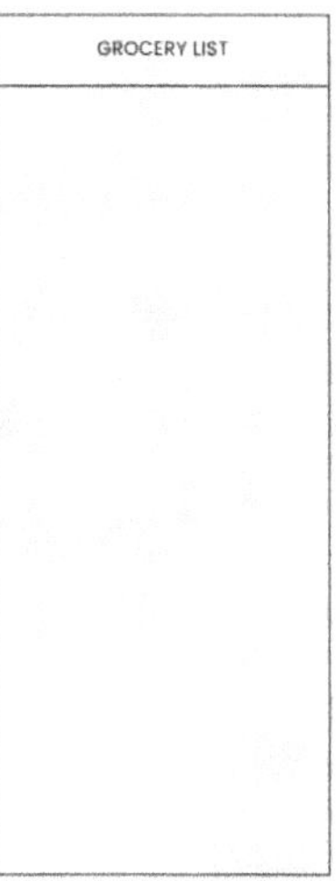
	LUNCH		
	DINNER		
TUESDAY	BREAKFAST		
	LUNCH		
	DINNER		
WEDNESDAY	BREAKFAST		
	LUNCH		
	DINNER		
THURSDAY	BREAKFAST		
	LUNCH		
	DINNER		
FRIDAY	BREAKFAST		
	LUNCH		SNACKS
	DINNER		
SARTURDAY	BREAKFAST		
	LUNCH		
	DINNER		
SUNDAY	BREAKFAST		
	LUNCH		
	DINNER		

WEEKLY MEAL PLANNER

MONDAY	BREAKFAST	
	LUNCH	
	DINNER	
TUESDAY	BREAKFAST	
	LUNCH	
	DINNER	
WEDNESDAY	BREAKFAST	
	LUNCH	
	DINNER	
THURSDAY	BREAKFAST	
	LUNCH	
	DINNER	
FRIDAY	BREAKFAST	
	LUNCH	
	DINNER	
SARTURDAY	BREAKFAST	
	LUNCH	
	DINNER	
SUNDAY	BREAKFAST	
	LUNCH	
	DINNER	

GROCERY LIST

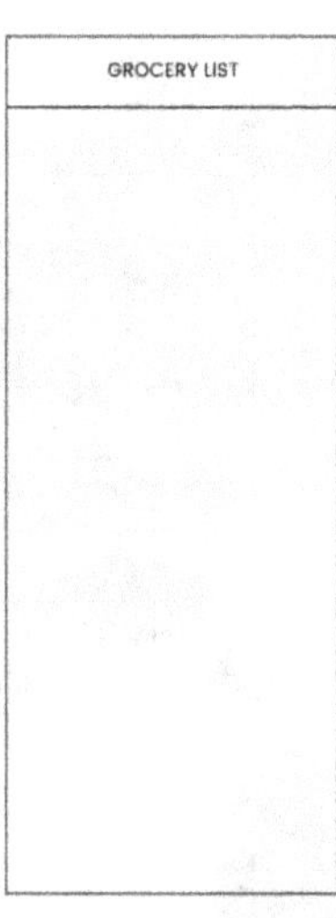

SNACKS

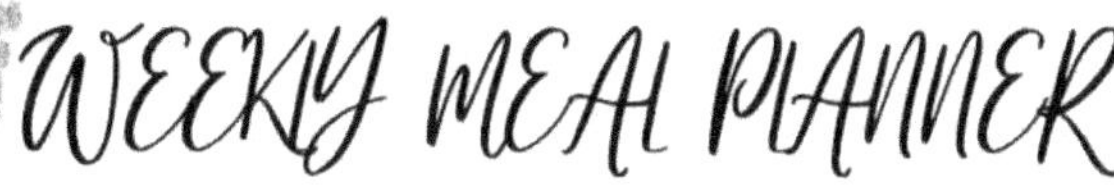

WEEKLY MEAL PLANNER

MONDAY	BREAKFAST	
	LUNCH	
	DINNER	
TUESDAY	BREAKFAST	
	LUNCH	
	DINNER	
WEDNESDAY	BREAKFAST	
	LUNCH	
	DINNER	
THURSDAY	BREAKFAST	
	LUNCH	
	DINNER	
FRIDAY	BREAKFAST	
	LUNCH	
	DINNER	
SARTURDAY	BREAKFAST	
	LUNCH	
	DINNER	
SUNDAY	BREAKFAST	
	LUNCH	
	DINNER	

GROCERY LIST

SNACKS

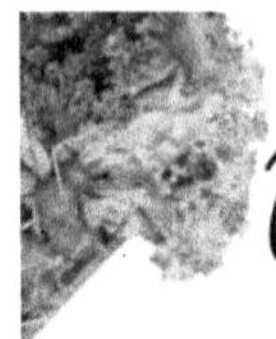

WEEKLY MEAL PLANNER

MONDAY	BREAKFAST	
	LUNCH	
	DINNER	
TUESDAY	BREAKFAST	
	LUNCH	
	DINNER	
WEDNESDAY	BREAKFAST	
	LUNCH	
	DINNER	
THURSDAY	BREAKFAST	
	LUNCH	
	DINNER	
FRIDAY	BREAKFAST	
	LUNCH	
	DINNER	
SARTURDAY	BREAKFAST	
	LUNCH	
	DINNER	
SUNDAY	BREAKFAST	
	LUNCH	
	DINNER	

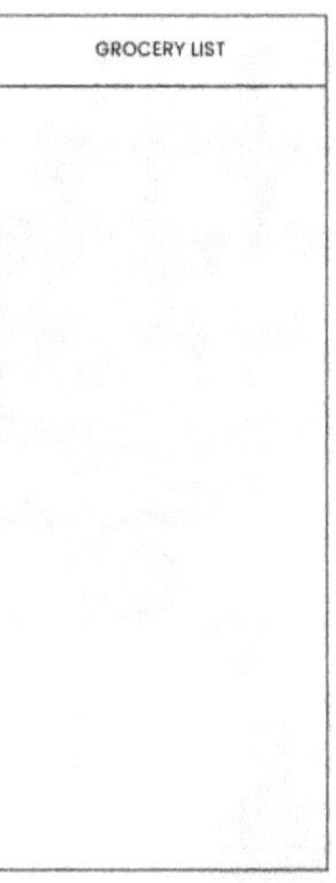

GROCERY LIST

SNACKS

www.ingramcontent.com/pod-product-compliance
Lightning Source LLC
Chambersburg PA
CBHW061645250726
48659CB00004B/1384